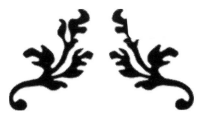

Condemned

by

Progressive Supranuclear Palsy

[Virulent Cousin of Parkinson's Disease]

J.F. Shepard

To Florence

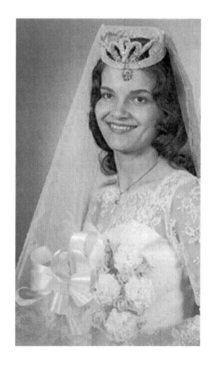

God Bless Her Beautiful
Soul

Published by Createspace, 4900 LaCross Rd.
Charleston, SC 29406

Additional Copies of this book available through
Amazon.Com

ISBN 10: 0-692-02709-2

ISBN 13: 978-0-692-02709-7

Library of Congress Control Number
2014906964

ACKNOWLEDGEMENTS

The author gratefully acknowledges the most valuable manuscript reviews by Dr. J.K. Uyemoto, Ph.D., and Dr. S. Chew, M.D. In addition, helpful suggestions by E. Calhoun and S. Hicks are recognized.

TABLE OF CONTENTS

CHAPTER 4 – HOSPICE CARE Ctd.

1

Prologue

There are very few books available that deal with the humanistic aspects of the *Progressive Supranuclear Palsy* disease (PSP) relevant to people caring for a relative or a friend sickened by the disease. The aim of this book is to acquaint, and offer insight to the reader into the dreadful process of this disease. Even so, this writing cannot be a step-by-step manual for those people dealing with PSP for the first time. Each patient may experience a different range, sequence, or intensity of symptoms (especially early on) or may respond uniquely to individual treatments making each caregiving task an individual endeavor. In this book, is the story of a tragedy, as are all premature deaths of a mother, but for it to take place over such a protracted period of suffering is particularly devastating. It also chronicles how in the absence of any prior caregiving experience, I coped with management of the disease from beginning to end for almost exactly eight years with my only legitimate personal goal being to make things as comfortable and pleasant as possible for my wife of 52 years during the final period of her life. This commemorative work is not expected to be a literary masterpiece, but instead it is intended to identify guideposts of disease progression and assist in the various steps of palliative care for physicians and caregivers dealing with PSP. If an element of information or comment included herein is discomforting in any aspect of the medical or other professional community, be assured that all situations described did occur and are accurately detailed.

THE DISEASE

Progressive Supranuclear Palsy (PSP) is a rare neuro-degenerative disorder of which few are aware, fewer have encountered; is never mentioned in daily media, and is the object of only a few national charities or research campaigns. The *CUREPSP Foundation for PSP, CBD and related Brain Diseases* is perhaps the most active advocate in the United States, and similar organizations exist in other countries. Nevertheless, lack of attention remains a major limitation for private or public reasearch funding at a time when other candidates in the Rare Diseases category, derive substantial research support. PSP is incurable and once a person is afflicted, life expectancy is reduced to an average of seven years with the time of survival somewhat dependent upon the quality of caregiving. It is to be expected that usually, the final two years in the patient's torment will be so uncomfortable, frustrating and depressing as to leave him/her little in the way of joy or zest for life. This book intends to give a voice to such people suffering from PSP (who can no longer speak for themselves) in hopes that some influential agency will listen.

In general, PSP causes permanent and serious motor skill problems including gait and balance, accompanied by an growing inability to aim the eyes upward or downward correctly. The disease's lengthy title implies that it begins slowly, continues to worsen (progressive) and causes weakness (palsy) from damage to certain pea-sized brain stem structures (called nuclei) in the brain, and it is here that higher-level (supra) control of eye movement degenerates and is ultimately lost.

This is a debilitating malady that is routinely confused with Parkinson's disease (PD), and it may also be incorrectly diagnosed as *Atypical Parkinson's Disease.* Such a conclusion is also misleading since the disease is, in fact, a different member of a group of related little-known brain disorders which also includes *Corticobasal Degeneration* (CBD), and *Multiple System Atrophy* (MSA) all of which lead to progressive decline. Ahlskog compared symptoms of PSP with those of PD in some detail and clearly identified differences between the two disorders. Symptom patterns of both do share some commonalities and early drug treatment for one, i.e., carbidopa/levodopa (carbo/levo) or *Sinemet,* may be somewhat effective for the other. But, in truth, PSP is a distinct malady; particular regions of the brain affected are not precisely the same as those involved in Parkinson's disorder. Like Parkinson's disease, PSP is a *Tauopathic* disease meaning that over production of a specific protein class (*Tau protein*) occurs in brainstem cells leading to their deterioration and the demise of nerve function. Affected are neurons controlling several key muscle groups including those governing muscles in arms, legs, face, eyes, and throat. Parenthetically, increased tau protein levels in the blood have also been correlated with damaging concussions in hockey players which reaffirms the involvement of this protein class in brain pathology.

TYPICAL SYMPTOMS OF PSP

Loss of normal equilibrium leading to frequent falls often (but not always) emerges as a regular problem at the onset of the disease. Psychological abnormalities emerge including anxiety, depression, apathy and withdrawal. Most facial expressions are compromised even under conditions which formerly provoked smiles, frowns and the like. An eventual classic sign of the disease is an inability to aim the eyes properly, especially downward at first and upward later on in the disease process. Eventually, mobility is completely lost, as is vision, and ability to swallow, eat, drink or talk. Arm and hand muscles contract generating a gnarled condition making the act of gripping impossible and painful to the touch. Because of the pain, no longer may you hold hands together. Some other signs include poor eyelid function, slow gait, impaired balance, a backward tilt of the head with stiffening of the neck muscles, sleep disruption (which at least in Florence's case predictably lead to temporary facial and upper extremity tremors), urinary incontinence and bowel irregularities.

A particular and enduring symptom class associated with PSP is *heightened anxiety* accompanied by *akathisia;* the latter of which is expressed as inner uneasiness or an antsy feeling often paired with an inability to sit still or get comfortable. A restless leg syndrome is also common. All elements of anxiety cause constant discomfort, unrest and stress to the patient throughout the duration of the disease. Successful treatment of this condition is difficult if not impossible to achieve. Carbo/levo can be helpful during early phases, and properly selected tranquilizers particularly when used in combination often provide psychological relief. Attempting to manage the condition is an unrelenting and ever changing task for the caregiver throughout the extent of the illness.

Unlike Parkinson's Disease, arm, hand or facial tremors are usually not an obvious or regular symptom in PSP, and another clear distinction between PSP and PD is the fact that premature death is always a predictable outcome in the former, but less frequently so in the latter. Despite all of this disheartening symptomatology, cognition, basic intelligence, hearing and memory may remain only lightly affected for some years in PSP, making life a living hell for a person who is often still aware enough to feel trapped in a failed body.

Once provoked, preliminary symptoms begin abruptly and then enter into an inexorably progressive phase of the PSP syndrome; viz., each symptom class worsens and additional types appear as times goes on. While a blank facial affect or problems with gait and balance coupled with dizziness may be the first signs of PSP, certain ensuing symptoms are classic and fully predictable at some point in the process.

- Expect that each and all symptoms or disorders will progressively worsen with time.
- No significant reduction in frequency or intensity of symptoms will be gained from administration of drugs save for transitory benefit from carbo/levo and anti-anxiety medications.
- No form of physical or occupational therapy will be of lasting benefit.
- Expect no sustained periods of remission as is sometimes observed in such other fatal diseases as cancer.

PSP was initially described as the *Steele-Richardson-Olszewski Syndrome* in 1963 to recognize the three Canadian physicians who first distinguished it from Parkinson's Disease. While deemed relatively rare (up to 2 victims per 100,000 or 20,000 people in the United States), the actual frequency may be as much as 30 percent higher due to misdiagnosis or when left undiagnosed in nursing homes or other senior facilities. Sadly, the rarity of the disease renders it unfamiliar to much of the medical community. Most primary care physicians, and many general neurologists have never seen it first-hand; frightening if you happen to be a victim. The condition afflicts both men and women and most (with exceptions) are affected at age 60 and above. Typically, a final diagnosis of the disorder takes up to four years which can further aggravate the problem because, in the interim, anti-Parkinson's drugs are often prescribed which may not only prove to be ineffective, but can also result in unpleasant and needless side-effects. From the time of onset, life spans are shortened to between five and eight years. It has often been put forth that of itself; PSP is not a fatal disease. Rather, it has been suggested that secondary factors are the primary cause of death and not the disease itself. If true this notion would seem encouraging to people during early phases of the disease once an accurate diagnosis is established. But, the idea is misleading. It is true that death frequently results from such secondary conditions as *Aspiration Pneumonia* (resulting from food "going down the wrong way"), head and other trauma from falls, or organ failure during the late phase "system shut-down". But, metaphorically, consider that a bullet fired from a gun of itself doesn't kill (as if by lead poisoning), but instead it inflicts damage which may lead to death even from such less direct causes as infection. Cause of death would still be gunshot! The same is true for PSP. The disease is predictably lethal whatever the culminating event might be. Numerous celebrities have suffered including the noted film actor Dudley Moore who died of this neurological horror in 2002 at age 66, American singer Teresa Brewer, who at 76 died from the effects of this disease in 2007, and very recently (April 2014) the Tony Award winning deaf actress, Phyllis Frelich, also succumbed to the disease.

What extrinsic factor(s) or molecular mechanism(s) trigger the onset of PSP is not established, and there is apparently little commonality within the pre-disease histories of one victim versus the next. Suggested possible causes include viral infection, genetic mutations or genetic related predisposition, chemical induction, and/or free radical cellular damage. None has been proven or been consistently observed. And later in this book, I will suggest that there is yet another potential cause.

CURRENT INFORMATION

It is not the objective of this book to offer an in-depth scientific or clinical treatise of PSP filled with pages upon pages of extensive medical jargon. That coverage may be found in the *Sourcebook* published by The National Institutes of Health and other publications (see the "Other Reading" section) along with a listing of PSP support groups may be quickly found through an online search. Another reference that should definitely be on the shelf of every neurologist is the clinical monograph, *Progressive Supranuclear Palsy Diagnosis, Pathology, and Therapy* by E. Tolosa et. al., 2013. This treatise offers the most up to date clinical and basic research in areas of PSP epidemiology, neuropathology, neurophysiology, and treatment.

Most current public information is in the form of on-line reports and flyers from major institutions such as the Mayo Clinic as well as from many other medical schools. But, be aware, several inconsistencies may be encountered in these articles because patients may well react differently especially during early stages of the disease. It is also true that some research reports may not have undergone peer review to guarantee accuracy.

THE VICTIM

The victim in this tragedy was a mother of two children and the grandmother of four. Her name was

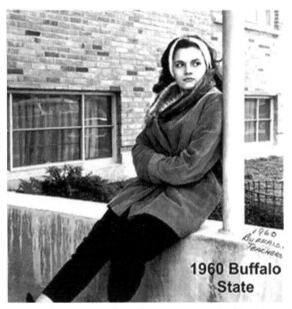

1960 Buffalo State

Florence, but most family members called her Flo, and at the onset of disease, she was 63 years of age and in excellent health. All of her vital signs including blood pressure, heart rate, blood sugar, cholesterol levels, etc. were enviable compared with equivalent readings of mine. Her hair was long, dark brown and had not been invaded by a single white strand. Even at this advanced age, her facial skin was soft and supple, totally free from wrinkles and called for no make-up save for a little eye liner. She stood a scant five foot three inches tall, but her small stature in no way suggested her to be a small person. Quite the contrary, Florence was considerate and gentle to all, possessed a big heart, and never spoke badly of any soul she encountered. In her youth, she was not popular with the boys and (as was true for me also) was left out of much of the activities of the socially elite in high school. She had to use any free hours for work, needing to contribute to family finances. She still found time to develop her admirable talent for drawing, painting and other forms of self-expression, and to put together a portfolio of her work. Though from a working class family, her parents did their best to assist her when she chose to enroll in the fine arts curriculum at Buffalo State College in Western New York State. She possessed an overwhelming desire to create, a quality than never abated throughout her entire life. Her character revealed itself in each of the beautiful oil paintings, pen and ink drawings, charcoal sketches, and water-colors she made over time. In addition, she created all manner of, needlework, including monogramming, and hand embroidered notices of each grandchild's arrival. All creations were done only as gifts to family and friends except for her fine quality monogramming which was commercially available. Florence would commonly devote much of her free time to her artistic activities and to her family. She was deeply loved by all who came to know her, including my five siblings who fully accepted her as sister number six. Truly a gift from God to this family.

After only one successful year, Florence left college to marry, discontinuing her formal education for 18 years upon which she matriculated in the school of architecture at Kansas State University. Like many of the artistic persuasion, by nature, she was introverted, shy and quiet around unfamiliar people and gentle among those she loved.

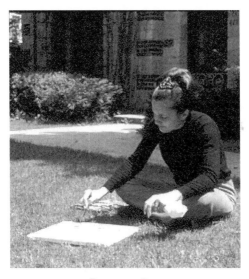

FLORENCE PAINTING

I hold an advanced college degree in a biological science, but I am not a medical doctor. Fortunately (depending upon how you look at it), I was retired throughout the

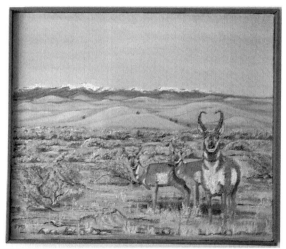

Three Montana Antelope by Florence Shepard

period of my wife's illness. Thus, I possessed sufficient scientific understanding to cope with many aspects of the disorder, and the time necessary to provide caregiving on a 24 hour basis. Of course, things would be quite different for another person serving as a primary caregiver who also had to hold a professional position or generate family income.

At present, there are still no curative or ameliorative drugs for PSP and few if any ever appeared on the most distant horizon. However, recently a promising clinical trial evaluated the publicized drug *Davunetide*, and while, initial results were promising enough for the FDA to put the drug on a "fast track" status for possible approval pending the outcome of large clinical trials. More on the subject of this drug will be presented later. So as difficult it is to accept, once PSP is accurately identified, it would seem to accomplish nothing (as we discovered) to go from one notable clinic to another frantically searching for a cure or at least meaningful treatment. What was needed most was effective medical counsel, and both physical and emotional support.

2

The Beginning

INTRA-ORAL PROSTHESIS

Yet another dental appointment for Florence. It was a clear, sunny but ominous Tuesday, October 18, 2005 as we made the short drive to the dental office. When a young person in a city with no fluoridation of drinking water, she suffered from innumerable dental caries (cavities), and consequently, as the years passed, some teeth were damaged beyond repair and removed. She was now at the point where some form of a three tooth bridge was needed to fill in a large gap between her right canine and rear molar. By this day, she had already undergone all of the needed processes of dental impressions, all other required steps, and now it was time to be fitted with the intra-oral prosthesis. A removable type was chosen over a fixed bridge for financial reasons, even though this option was preferred by neither of us (and we were soon to regret the choice). As the mouthpiece was unpackaged, we were surprised to find that the plate (which was designed by an affiliated dental prosthesis manufacturing company) was constructed with a large metal amalgam base rather than having been fabricated solely with resin composites as we had expected. Despite our concerns, her dentist, Dr. Schmidt, assured us that all would be well as he made final adjustments and inserted the device. When finished, he escorted us to the checkout desk and once again assured us that Florence would get used to the

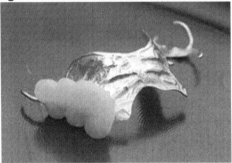

Problematic Prosthesis

fit. After just a few days, Florence was uncomfortable with the mouthpiece; the fit was too tight, and her gums were so irritated that she could only tolerate the prosthesis during brief periods when she was out in public. In January of 2006, we had a follow-up session after earlier complaining about the fit to Dr. Schmidt. He adjusted the mouthpiece a bit and then advised her to wear it regularly. If she did not, he cautioned, natural changes in tooth alignment over time would alter the fit and render the partial plate worthless. So in it went by day, but at night, it was removed and soaked in dilute mouthwash or water. Within two, weeks (mid-February), Florence began to negatively react to the prosthesis. Gums became inflamed, and both throat and face swelled as if there was a hypersensitive reaction of some kind. The condition could go on no longer! Of necessity, use of the $2,000 plate was completely discontinued, after which facial swelling began to recede. We were suspicious that the amalgam base may have contributed to the problem, and we asked her primary physician to order blood tests for heavy metals. He did so, but no abnormality was detected.

The Beginning   21

APPEARANCE OF INITIAL PSP SYMPTOMS

By March 7, 2006, Florence's face was no longer swollen, a good thing we thought, but, surprisingly, her face had assumed a permanent look of indifference regardless of the momentary circumstance (termed *blank affect* or *masked condition*). It seemed that either she had lost the absolute ability to develop a smile, had relinquished any desire to do so, or both. Concomitantly, there was a noticeable change in her emotional condition. While her face physically suggested apathy, she also appeared to have become emotionally detached. No longer did she show interest in events that once were constantly on her mind such as family member birthdays, what meals to prepare, what to shop for, any form of humor, etc.

I personally maintain a large cactus collection in a small greenhouse and all members of the collection are famous for their spectacular blooms during late spring and summer. Before her illness, Florence was gleeful upon the appearance of each and every flower. In early spring, she anxiously awaited emergence of her most favorite flower, the hyacinth. She loved them all and it was always uplifting to me to witness her joy as they burst into bloom. But, with the sudden loss of emotion, Florence became totally indifferent to the the lovely blooms and even ceased visiting the our cactus greenhouse. For a time, the symptoms were very frustrating for me because I had never encountered anything like them before. I was confused by her abnormal behavior and had no idea of its cause. Only much later did I finally come to know the nature and origin of the problem.

As if the facial and emotional symptoms were not enough for her to suffer through, she was also constantly dizzy, suffered from an uninterrupted ringing in her ears (*tinnitus*) and generally felt unsteady. I expect that all of us have dealt with each of these symptoms individually for a short while, but try to imagine what it would be like for all three types occurring at once, permanently. She must have been very miserable, but true to her nature, there was little in the way of a prolonged complaint from her.

SEARCH FOR A CAUSE

Day to day life was becoming so intolerable for Florence that we were forced to make repeated visits to her primary physician in hopes that some improvement in her status might be realized. None of us knew at the time how rare the affliction was, or its origin, and we failed to recognize how few physicians were either aware of it or had any knowledge of how to treat it. Our primary physician ordered a cranial Magnetic Resonance Imaging (MRI) which when analyzed showed no obvious abnormality or tumor. We were frightened, confused and lacked direction. It seemed clear to us that the ill-conceived dental piece was behind the problem despite an absence of definitive proof. We asked the primary care physician to refer us to a professional who would be familiar enough with the symptoms we had observed to this point to give guidance and treatment. Presumably, the most qualified specialist to this end would be a neurologist; a physician dealing with disorders of the nervous system. We were referred to a physician we will call Neurologist #1, a member of a good sized neurology group of some local repute, who was located nearby in the

Doctor's Annex of a large hospital. This chap was a husky, gray haired man with a lined face in his late 60's wearing rumpled clothes and a bow tie. Right off, I was not at ease with him and was cautious when I spoke to avoid agitating him. He had immigrated from Germany in the late 1950's and was quite decided in his opinions; those relating to this examination and just about everything else including strong negative views on the field of stem cell research. His justification, "I don't want scientists to keep killing babies!" A bit obtuse for a physician since, to most people, stem cell research seems to offer great potential in neurology. I reminded him (or perhaps informed him) that most stem cell lines these days were no longer sourced from human embryos. Overall, he was a person easily put off by; no master of discourse, never a smile and no signs of compassion, concern, or understanding. Immediately I was doubtful that any worthwhile prospects would emerge from this visit. We wound up settling for him, briefly, because the head of his neurology group (who we originally requested) was no longer taking new patients. While we were there, Neurologist #1 performed the usual (in retrospect) cursory walk-a-line (for *ataxia*) and eye movement (for *nystagmus*) tests (akin to a field sobriety test – hereafter referred to as the *DUI test*). His conclusion; "Yes indeed, Florence definitely has a problem with her balance." His diagnosis; "The cause is most probably an inner ear infection, and I will refer you to an excellent specialist." As we left his office, Florence and I were both skeptical that an inner ear infection was the source of the disorder, but to cover all avenues, off we went to a respected Ear, Nose and Throat (ENT) specialist. Following a complete battery of tests concerning hearing level, function, and health, ENT analysis found no inner ear infection problems nor any other hearing discrepancy.

Dizziness plus the masked facial condition persisted and we were becoming increasingly frustrated with not knowing the cause. No physician we had visited, to date, had offered any form of believable diagnosis or prognosis, and we were at loss as to what should be our next move. I contacted my youngest sister Mary, a nurse with many years' experience in geriatric care. She immediately flew out from Rochester, New York, and requested a visit with the primary care physician. Mary had not seen this particular syndrome, but there were similarities including masking among some of her patients. She suggested that something should immediately be tried to control the dizziness. *Dramamine* and a few other anti-motion sickness drugs were tested after consultation with our primary care physician, but either they did little to improve her vertigo, were ineffective, or simply acted through sedation. Hence, all proved of little value. In retrospect, I must admit, however, even if such an approach might be viewed as naive, many other motion sickness or anti-nausea drugs (such as *Ondansetron, Diazepam, Phenergan* and/or *Stugeron*) should also have been tested for efficacy. Any drug that would have eased her distress would have been most beneficial.

Florence had always been quite sensitive or hypersensitive to medications of all sorts, and each new one had to be carefully tested for abnormal reactions before repeated use. Many years ago she nearly died from inept (without testing for sensitivity) administration of *Succinylcholine* during tubal ligation surgery. Within seconds, she experienced a hypersensitive reaction and stopped breathing. It was all the staff could do to stabilize her. This served as a dramatic warning that any new medications must be judiciously tested prior to dosing.

And, as we shall see later, with this knowledge in hand, we sometimes were not alert enough.

Even at this early stage in the disease, Florence was nearly always dizzy with constantly ringing in her ears. She wrote to my sister on May 4, 2006;

"Thank you for your thoughts. I appreciate your motivational emails. I need to make another doctor's appointment for a check-up. I don't really want to do it as I think he will send me for a CAT scan or an MRI. My ears have been ringing, and I am dizzy a lot and get easily confused. I forget a lot. Jim has had it with me and I don't blame him."

It was true, regrettably, that I was often short on patience during those early phases. For some reason, I had neither accepted nor fully appreciated the fact that when she was slow in gait or response, it was this unknown condition that was at fault not her frame of mind or intent. While she was still mentally acute, it, nonetheless, took longer now for her to formulate a response before she would speak. Indeed, on one of my especially inconsiderate days, I likened her slow walk to that portrayed by a stricken person in an episode of the TV series *Night Court* who was said, by Dan, to have *Tortoise Nervosa*. I found that comment funny, Florence did not, and in time I would come to understand that comments regarding a slow gait or any other of her symptoms were not suitable material as jokes.

PSP PROGRESSION

In many cases of PSP, loss of balance occurs after a patient's head suddenly tilts backward or unexpectedly sideways. It has been reported that these types of fall are a frequent preliminary symptom in disease development, sometimes even during the very initial phases. Such was not true for Florence. Side effects of her irregular balance and diminished coordination meant that there were things she could no longer do, like safely driving an automobile, but even infrequent falls, though seemingly inevitable, did not begin to occur throughout 2006. However, during this time, there was a decline in the quality of her penmanship. Previously, her writing was always lovely and clearly out shined my efforts, but, that was beginning to change.

Through all of this, Florence showed no signs of dementia and seemed to be fully cognizant of the situations around her. She was also otherwise very healthy. Her appetite was good, and vital signs including blood pressure, heart rate, blood sugar and cholesterol levels, triglycerides, etc. remained in ideal ranges. Even so, her senses were not quite as sharp as before, and a longer period of time was needed for her to respond to stimuli. She continued to maintain her household routine as best as she could. One day she unexpectedly began to furiously pack personal belongings from about the house into storage bins, almost at random, like a squirrel burying a store of winter acorns. Many of my personal favorites like gloves, hunting clothes, and other odd things abruptly disappeared into unmarked bins. Kitchen towels, sheets, pillowcases, became in short supply. Strange indeed, and despite my complaining, she could not forestall the urge.

During 2006 and into 2007, Florence attempted to prepare our favorite dishes for lunch and dinner. But, as time progressed, such tasks were increasingly difficult because of balance issues. One day she made baked custard, an item always on the top of my favorite homemade dessert list. When baking was complete, she did not inform me that she needed help, but instead attempted to remove the heavy crockery dish from the oven on her own. It slipped from her hands, and custard spilled all across the kitchen floor leaving nothing in the dish. She wept uncontrollably for a time, not only because of the loss of custard, but also because she clearly recognized that she was losing control of the muscles in her hands. "What is to become of me," she sobbed, "I just couldn't hold on to it." I felt so sorry for her as I cleaned up

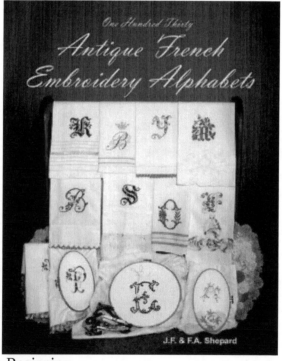

remnants of the dish. She always had made the finest custard that I ever tasted, including that of my mother, but, at this point, that treat had sadly become a thing of the past.

We still continued trying to engage in activities that we always enjoyed together like visiting antique shops, grocery shopping, and taking in quaint nearby towns on weekends. The pace of our movements were, of necessity, much slower than before, but we still managed. I always walked close to help steady her or hand in hand. We had always spent most all of our free and, in business time together as a couple. For twenty five years, we owned our own businesses and worked throughout each day with one another. We had travelled a great deal, took many cruises, and visited the Amazon River along with other delightful destinations. We wanted to continue doing things but, were beginning to fear that the "activities" aspect of our marriage would soon need to be curtailed. Florence became very worried but typically she internalized much of her anguish. She had been an excellent artist and in earlier times did many oil and watercolor paintings. Working with her hands, and doing crafts was her great passion. As mentioned earlier, she was an expert with a sewing needle and created hundreds of monogrammed linens both for sale and for gifts to family and friends. Evidence of her skill may be seen on the front cover of our book, *One Hundred Thirty Antique French Embroidery Alphabets* where monogrammed letters from eleven different antique alphabets done by her are on display. She was also accomplished with tatting, crocheting, and knitting as well as other types of embroidery. But, the needlework examples shown on the book cover were the last she was physically able to do. In her near expressionless face, I could still see fear in her dark brown eyes; fear that she might never again be able to engage in any of her favorite skills.

SEARCH FOR A NEUROLOGIST

We were less than satisfied with the "findings" of Neurologist #1, and in response to our pleading, our primary physician referred us to a second specialist, hereafter known as Neurologist #2. After a 45 minute drive, we finally found his office located in one corner of a building used by a local television station. We were greeted at his office by a clerk who demanded a high co-payment which I grudgingly paid. This doctor was in his forties, short, portly, bald headed, and quite straight forward. He informed us that he could only allow us a brief get acquainted visit until he conducted an MRI (he owned his own diagnostic equipment). We argued that we had very recently had an MRI done and that we would have the films sent to him posthaste. Thereafter, he performed the standard DUI test but was uncertain what to make of it. Coolly, he agreed to set another appointment once the MRI films arrived. (Things are much more convenient today, of course, and images may be carried about on a CD).

One week later we returned, presented our co-pay, and were directed to an examination room, whereupon were advised that the doctor would soon be with us. Abruptly, before we were even seated, the doctor entered the room and stated that he could come to no conclusions from viewing the MRI and determined that he could not be of help. However, he agreed to assist us in making an appointment (referral required) with Neurologist #3 who was purportedly the most qualified M.D. in the region having won renown for geriatric neurological problems. He authored many relevant scientific publications, and headed a university hospital center for aged neurology including such disorders as Parkinsonism. But, he apparently was so busy doing one thing or another that we were forced to wait six months for an appointment.

When we met Neurologist #3, we were truly hopeful of getting help for Florence's worsening condition. The physician viewed the MRI films we brought, and conducted the usual DUI test. From these observations and other facts from his interview, he concluded that Florence was most likely suffering from early stages of Parkinson's disease (PD). Accordingly, he prescribed *Sinemet* (carbo/levo), a standard medication for PD. Once taken, carbo/levo did prove to be of some benefit to her. Dizziness, though still present, was a little reduced and balance was slightly improved. The first thing in the morning she would say, "I need my Sinemet to get my heart started". While not a panacea, it was true that Sinemet administration seemed effective in transmitting mental commands to her lethargic muscles. Despite these transitory benefits, anxiety level was exacerbated by the constant administration of carbo/levo, and we were forced to search for a compensating tranquilizer(s).

For now, we at least had a lead (if you wish to call it that). The first two neurologists were of no help, and apparently were unable to recognize this neurological disorder altogether. Now with the conclusion of Neurologist #3 that Parkinson's disease was a possibility, Florence and I purchased a number of popular and scientific books on the subject and read avidly. If the disease was, in fact, PD, at least it should be manageable. Lots of people have PD! We then attempted to make a follow-up appointment with Neurologist #3 to discuss subjects such as progressive anxiety, and physical instability to name a few. No luck! We would have to wait for seven months before he would be available for a follow-up appointment and even that date was subject to change. Apparently, he had a number of national meetings to attend, awards to receive, and the like with little time left over to care for his patients. And, despite being the chairman of a clinic for geriatric neurology, we were told that no other physician in his clinic was qualified to treat Florence. Some clinic! The situation was totally unacceptable! My goal was to find a neurologist well-schooled in PD who was available for assisting us on a regular basis, not once or twice a year.

TRYING TO COPE

Over the next several months, other physical anomalies began to appear. Her neck muscles were in constant spasm causing neck stiffness and pain. To help alleviate some of this discomfort, physicians at a pain clinic in Kansas City, performed *Facet Joint Injections* of a steroid into inflamed spinal joints at the base of the skull. This procedure was successful in moderating the level of neck and shoulder pain but, it did little to reduce stiffness. During this time, the quality of her handwriting, once superb, further deteriorated and was beginning to be difficult for me to read. Irregular sleep patterns along with heightened anxiety, and frequent tossing and turning during the night made sleep difficult for her. Occasional minor falls took place around the house, but none was serious. Thank goodness that, at that time, we did not have hardwood floors in the house. Universal carpeting saved her from considerable injury. When falls did occur, most happened when Florence was rising from a chair or bed. To reduce the risk of a serious tumble, an electric lift chair was purchased making it easier for her to rise from a chair without the risk of falling. Over time, the constancy and severity of her anxiety increased and her physical coordination declined. Her eyes became especially sensitive to bright light and when out of doors, dark wrap-around sunglasses were mandatory even on cloudy days. And, in the house, when we moved her about in a wheel chair, sunglasses were required if we located her near the sliding glass doors or under bright kitchen lights.

By the middle of 2007, two years into the syndrome, we wondered what our next steps should be. It had now been years of medical confusion with little if any assistance. All that I was able to do was to perform palliative care accompanied by a lot of guess work as each symptom appeared. There was no reference book to consult, nor a physician with ready answers. Thank goodness Florence was such an accommodating patient who willingly agreed to whatever I proposed so long as it seemed reasonable. She was taking the maximum recommended carbo/levo doses at four hour intervals daily and was also sequentially prescribed additional tranquilizers in an attempt to calm the exacerbating effects of carbo/levo on her anxiety. However, neither *Xanax* alone nor other promising candidates tested proved satisfactory which left Florence uncomfortable and hyperactive as if on a constant verge of a panic attack. She complained of a restless leg syndrome along with the other symptoms.

About this point, my family and I naively thought that Florence might enjoy spending time in a senior activity center which specializes in caring for mentally or physically disabled persons. After much searching, we identified a suitable facility which would even pick Florence up and return her home at night. Various activities were offered throughout the day to keep patients occupied. Florence said that she would be willing to go to the "home" if I wished, but her counsel was of little value because she was always worried that I was working too hard and would agree to most anything if it was for my benefit. After a bit of time, I concluded that the true underlying cause for my search was aimed at selfishly reducing my caregiving load. In reality, Florence was too ill even to sit up all day, and would not enjoy the company of other people at this point. When lucidity returned to me, I reckoned that she could only be happy at home.

As we went along, I often wondered what form of terror must be going on in her mind. In the earlier times, she would say that she was uncomfortably woozy most all of the time. Imagine how unpleasant that condition would be, and how the sensation would interfere with our normal responses. Especially when despite dizziness, ancillary pain, and other problems, the person is fully cognizant of events surrounding them. No surprise that a PSP patient typically exhibits a progressive personality change and generally becomes indifferent. Who wouldn't be when suffering from multiple types of mental discomfort day and night. Later on, as additional symptoms appeared and her overall physical condition declined, she still was unable to describe, fully, how she felt - apart from the statement; "I feel trapped in a dysfunctional body almost as if I am claustrophobic for no reason." Through it all, she found comfort from her relationship with her mother who at that time was 85 years old. She lived alone in a senior apartment in central Kansas, and while she was able to drive her car locally, the two and one half hour trip to our home was to frightening for her take on by herself. Thus, my son and I shared driving duties on special holidays and at other times through the year to facilitate her visits. These were always special times for Florence. Earlier she wrote,

"My mother is an inspiration to me. She exercises three times a week, goes line dancing often and participates in a senior center in Junction City. She also takes care of a little dog which entails walks outside and lots of maintenance plus a cat. I am twenty years younger and haven't nearly the energy that my mother has. She has always inspired me. In my teenage years when I was learning to drive, I was ready to quit, but she would not let me because she had learned to drive and couldn't imagine living without being able to get herself around. She is an independent person and she has tried to make me independent as well. Nobody wants to take care of someone else so you have to learn to care for yourself. My mother is a living example of that fact and has taken care of herself for some 85 years."

Throughout our married life, I was always perplexed by the fact that while Florence could express herself comfortably through her painting, handwork and writing, she was generally at a loss when attempting to express herself verbally on a sensitive issue. Sometimes I would ask her to write a response if that would make understanding easier, which she did on occasion. But now, with handwriting failing, and her recent inability to operate the keyboard of her computer, understanding her attempts at communication were becoming most difficult for me, and extraordinarily frustrating for her

Following the suggestion of Neurologist #3 that Parkinson's disease was the suspect, Florence voraciously read *The Parkinson's Disease Treatment Book* by J.E. Ahlskog, an excellent PD resource, in hopes of discovering useful suggestions and gaining an understanding of the prognosis. She was especially encouraged by the first two lines of text which read, *Parkinson's disease (PD) is a treatable condition. Medical treatment increases longevity and allows most people with PD to remain active and productive for many years.*

For Florence, many primary Parkinson's like symptoms were beginning to appear including trouble standing up, slow movement, facial masking, stiffness and asymmetric mobility, softer monotone voice, and a demise of autonomic movements like gesturing when talking and others. A major exception from the PD syndrome was the fact that *classic rest tremors* in face, arm or leg were absent. This was a clue for later on. On the basis of what we had heard, seen, and read to this point, we nonetheless proceeded under the PD premise with no awareness whatsoever of a disease called Progressive Supranuclear Palsy.

PHYSICAL THERAPY

It seemed logical to us and to others we consulted with that physical exercise might be useful to keep muscles toned and of potential value in maintaining proper balance. Our Humana Medicare Advantage Insurance program offers support for a physical fitness program to senior members called Silver Sneakers which is offered through a number of local physical fitness facilities. Florence joined this program through a nearby YMCA. This was an outstanding organization with a broad range of well-designed programs, excellent facilities, and fine instructors. Florence thoroughly enjoyed her periods of exercise two days a week along with an additional Yoga program on Fridays. Each day she enthusiastically filled her gym bag with requisite towels, socks, shorts, etc. and was at the door ready to go, generally a bit early. For each session, I would drive her to the facility and wait for an hour or so for her to complete the routine. She continued these programs for several months and was inspired by both the routines and the people. She met several nice folks in the process and looked forward to interactions with them at each session. Each day after the physical therapy session, Florence would recount a cute story she had heard from the group as I drove her home. More than anything, her sessions were most helpful for her mental state and attitude. While still unable to smile, there was a glint in her eyes, a rewarding thing to see. Though she felt that her programs were helpful in maintaining some stability, in the long run, it did little to stave off the inevitable loss of muscle control. Then, both unexpectedly and unfortunately, new rules were enacted at the YMCA whereby should any senior person undergo a fall during an exercise program, no matter how minor, the individual must be immediately transported to a hospital emergency room by ambulance to be checked out. Given the degree of her instability, the potential risk of this YMCA policy was financially too great for us to chance. An ambulance ride could cost $500 even with insurance. Sadly, Florence was forced to leave the Silver Sneakers program. There were no remaining external physical therapy programs available for people in her condition, and she no longer benefit from the human interaction she enjoyed so much. Hard and fast rules are obviously necessary to satisfy insurance company demands, but many people are destined to fall though the proverbial "crack." Sad indeed for *Crackees* like Florence who held no other real form of joy.

3

PHASE II

NEUROLOGICAL PING PONG

It was now June of 2008. For two plus years we had been bounced about from one physician to the next in the form of *neurological ping pong* with little if any professional progress or insight into Florence's problem. My eldest sister from St Louis was very concerned about our lack of care, and was familiar with yet another neurologist at a nearby prestigious research hospital whom she held in high regard. We agreed with her suggestion that a visit with him might well be worthwhile. We will refer to him as Neurologist #4.

From the literature and my personal observation of Florence's symptoms (which were not typical of those found in PD), I began to suspect that she was suffering from PSP rather than PD. I hoped that Neurologist #4 would provide a definitive answer to this question and would outline a beneficial course of treatment irrespective of what the ailment was because we were still not sure. From Kansas City, it was a four hour drive to the hospital in St. Louis, and we all hoped this lengthy trip would be worthwhile. It was a sunny morning, and we were both enjoying the drive together. It had been a long time since we shared any trip of more than 30 minutes. As we approached the hospital we were struck by its imposing size, and style. It was magisterial, a structure that subliminally promised healing just from its architectural form. Oh, if only this were true! We pulled into the underground parking facility, and I assisted Florence as she made her way through the doors to the elevators. Upon arriving at the 7th floor, we wandered around a bit and found the correct suite number. Soon after entry, we were greeted by the doctor at reception, not a common thing for physicians to do, and guided to his office. We were immediately impressed. He was a tall, elderly gentleman with both a high intellect and genuine concern for his patients, both unique qualities in our experience. His non-aggressive manner and gentle voice lent a calming effect to his us even though he was a bit inclined toward prolixity (verbose).

During the obligatory DUI exam, Neurologist #4 paid particular attention to Florence's eye movements. From this, he concluded that Florence was suffering from *Atypical Parkinson's Disease* and not PSP. He stated that to verify the disease as being PSP, downward eye movement and peripheral vision must be greatly inhibited while these symptoms are less apparent in PD. At this stage of disease development, Florence's downward eye control was only marginally abnormal. And, he justified this point in a lengthy treatise to defend the Atypical PD conclusion. The said write-up was transmitted to our primary physician and inserted into Florence's thick medical records file. I was surprised to learn that this portfolio was not available to me without written approval from Neurologist #4 who, for some reason only known to him, would never agree to provide the necessary signature. To some extent, the notion that Florence was suffering from Parkinson's disease was encouraging to hear because, if true, the prognosis would be better than if the disease were PSP. If PD, there need not be total immobility, not an early death and not the loss of eyesight, and other basic functions over the same period of time. On the return trip home, she was upbeat, feeling that if PD was her affliction, at least she should gain some benefit from drugs, and the promise of new drugs to treat PD was always there. I didn't contradict her or dampen her optimism, but, personally, I was not convinced of the diagnosis of Neurologist #4, and I feared that there would be no real benefit from this visit other than the possible positive effects of another anti-anxiety drug, *Zoloft,* that he had prescribed. The original carbo/levo dosage was left unchanged. At the doctor's request, we returned for a follow-up examination a few months later, but his opinion (diagnosis) was unaltered, and since we received nothing new in terms of treatment ideas, we decided not to return.

So here we were once again, reminiscent of the movie "Groundhog Day" where prior events kept repeating themselves. No convincing diagnosis, no encouraging prognosis, but unlimited obfuscation (mumbo jumbo). As months went by, Florence's balance disorder worsened and wooziness persisted. She said that life for her was like continually riding a small cruise ship on rough seas. We never found a medication that ameliorated that or her dizziness.

I still believed, naively, that there must be a neurologist out there somewhere who could provide us with genuine assistance, who could slow or stop the progression of symptoms. Long distance attempts had not been rewarding, so our search continued. By scanning the list of nearby neurology groups, I selected yet another physician, and we made an appointment in July of 2009. We hoped that he was worth the price since he accepted neither Medicare nor Medicare Advantage Insurance making the office call more expensive for us. We shall call him Neurologist #5. After reviewing her history, he performed the DUI test and came to a rapid bittersweet conclusion, "I believe Florence has PSP, not Parkinson's disease." By now her inability to move her eyes downward or to focus them properly had advanced to the point where he was quite certain of his diagnosis. Obviously, such a conclusion was subjective, but one which I had long suspected. It is amazing to me that a single symptom category, improper eye control, was needed to make a PSP diagnosis. Unfortunately, he followed the diagnosis with the statement, "There is nothing I can do for her. As things progress, if you need to refill any prescriptions or get new ones designed to make her more comfortable, don't hesitate to phone my office." So now we had an official confirmation of the disease right on cue. It had taken about four years of disease progression before the PSP diagnosis was made. But, the diagnosis was followed by the predictable statement, "I can do nothing for her, but come back in six months." I had heard that phrase from each neurologist. My immediate thought was, "Why?" No point in repeatedly going to a "specialist" who can offer no help, and is unwilling or unable to suggest another physician (we requested such) who would be more qualified and/or helpful. After five trials, I completely gave up on the neurology community in deference to handling situations on my own with assistance from the hospice personnel. I and my hospice crew apparently knew more about handling the PSP syndrome than any of the neurologists we had met; including how to treat it, and generally what palliative steps were needed on behalf of the patient under a plethora of circumstances.

ATTITUDE ADJUSTMENT

After abandoning any hope of assistance from the neurological profession, I decided that perhaps a change of scenery might exert a positive effect on Florence's attitude. She was beginning to suffer more and more by now both physically and mentally. It must have been very hard for her to acknowledge what was certainly in her future and still maintain a positive attitude. But, she never discussed such feelings with me or complained about her condition. By now, she was well aware that unlike PD, PSP was a terminal affliction and that further physical decline was inevitable.

Another of my sisters lives near Yosemite National Park in California. Travel was still possible for Florence so long as I pushed her about airports, etc. in a wheelchair. Walking for her, though still possible, was difficult, especially over long distances or if we were in a hurry. Balance and slow gait were the primary obstacles, while pain was yet to become of major significance. Off we went to California in September 2009, and my sister was a wonderful hostess for what proved to be Florence's last get away. In spite of the fires that devastated many parts of Yosemite in 2009, a delightful time was had touring

Yosemite Park including a sumptuous lunch at the Ahwahnee Hotel Dining Room. We moved on for two days at a Squaw Valley Village condo from which we circled Lake Tahoe and dined at several lovely lakeside restaurants. From there, we toured the fascinating ghost town of Bodie, California, alkaline Mono Lake with its fascinating tufa towers, and drove along the eastern side of the magnificent Sierra Nevada Mountains. After a forgettable night in the town of Lee Vining, on we went to Virginia City, Nevada with its generous slot machines in the *Bucket of Blood* saloon, very bumpy stagecoach rides and interesting silver mine tours. What a wonderful tour and Florence enjoyed it immensely, despite her difficulties in getting around by herself. Photographs taken during the trip revealed to me that Florence was no longer able to form a true smile and her head was commonly tilted

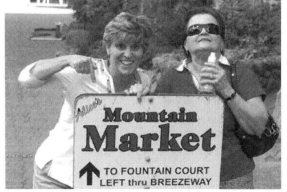

backward as seen here (on the right). This had been true to some extent from the beginning as a part of her masking problem. But here, her expression was more of a grimace with her face slightly contorted almost as if in pain, and she was beginning to need constant steadying while walking. Wheelchairs were used where possible as we focused on getting about and taking in as much as possible during our all too brief seven day visit.

The sad truth of vacations is that, upon your return home, you must again deal with the same problems that existed before hand plus having to cope with any additional ones that may have cropped up in your absence. As Barry McGuire once sang in his hit tune *Eve of Destruction*; *"You may leave here for four days in space, but when you return it's the same old place."*

RETURN TO REALITY

Once back from California, Florence underwent a noticeable decline. She started to suffer from sporadic urinary incontinence. At first panty liners helped control the condition, but as time wore on, senior briefs (like *Depends*) were needed. Of course, Florence was embarrassed by this and tried to both control and hide its occurrence as best she could. To this point in the disease progression, it is important to stress that the occurrence of any abnormal physical acts whether they relate to falling down, toileting, flopping into chairs or onto beds or lack of either facial expression or enthusiasm upon receipt of good news, is strictly attributable to the disease and were not the product of a conscious act by the afflicted person. In retrospect, this seems to be an obvious fact, but, when living the experience, any caregiver's patience will be sorely tested, often several times a day, and one is inclined to accuse the patient of being careless, or of behaving in such a way as to garner more attention, or of having no concern for the caregiver, etc., etc., and blah, blah, blah. Such ridiculous and thoughtless behavior by the caregiver can injure the already damaged and very fragile pride of the patient. I speak to this from experience and regret every incident of which I was guilty. One should always try to remember who the person was before the illness, and how much **they** long to be the same way again.

HOME HEALTH CARE

When independent exercise in public facilities became no longer possible, we then turned to the possibility of a home therapy program in an attempt to maintain muscle and mental tone. We discovered that, for those people 65 and older, Medicare supports home health with supplies under a defined system of bundled services. To qualify for home healthcare, a person must first be classified as "Homebound." Homebound in this case is defined as being *confined to the home* or being unable to leave without an immense effort. Persons may still be considered homebound if they only leave the home occasionally for short periods of time or for medical appointments. Such bundled services include:

- Skilled nursing visits
- Home health aide services
- Physical therapy
- Occupational therapy
- Covered routine medical supplies
- Medical social services

Administration by a licensed home health agency is required to qualify for Medicare coverage and a willing primary care physician must be designated to oversee the program.

We spoke with several home health companies, each presented relevant programs, and from this, we chose a respected local franchise. A physical therapy program was soon arranged, and a senior therapist devised a thorough physical training sequence which was to continue over a period of nine months. She, the therapist, seemed committed to Florence and worked hard to strengthen weakened muscles and worked diligently to improve stability. One to two hour sessions were held three days a week, and though they required considerable physical effort, Florence looked forward to each one.

Home care therapy also includes the services of an occupational therapist. Occupational therapy is skilled treatment that aims to "assist individuals in achieving independence in all facets of their lives". Occupational therapy presumes to provide people with the "skills for the job of living." According to Mayo School of Health Sciences, Occupational therapy services typically include:

- Customized treatment programs aimed at improving abilities to carry out the activities of daily living
- Comprehensive evaluation of home and job environments and recommendations on necessary adaptation
- Assessments and treatment for performance skills
- Recommendations and training in the use of adaptive equipment
- Guidance to family members and caregivers

Medicare supported our home health care program for three cycles of ninety days each, and sufficient "progress" was demonstrated for all of the critical physical therapy milestones. In truth, Florence did seem to measure up to each physical strength criterion during reviews, but, clearly, no progress was recorded in her level of stability. Various walking cane types were tested to determine whether they might aid in fall prevention. We tried canes with one, two and four feet, but all proved to be of no major benefit. She was particularly vulnerable to backward falls and canes were of little use in preventing these. Several walkers were then tried, and while backward falls were reduced, sideways falls were still frequent thus making it very risky for Florence to attempt to walk without human assistance.

While appreciating the efforts of the physical therapist, I was confused on the actual *raison d'être* of the occupational therapist. She offered suggestions on how the remove in home hazards that encouraged falls such as throw rugs, how to add hand-holds in critical places, how to set up the shower, and the like. Much attention was also directed toward the psychological aspects of the disease on the patient as well as caregiver. Nebulous suggestions and confusing directives were put forth in an attempt to correct our putative lack of dutiful friends willing to jump-in and assist caregiving at the drop of a hat. For example, I should become more active in church activities, should join this club or that, etc. I found little use for most of this. I did not want to leave Florence alone for long periods of time to do such things, and it was my experience during my parent's illnesses that friends and neighbors and even family members feel awkward, perhaps get a little bored around seriously sick people, and eventually withdraw.

In a recent University of Florida on-line research note, Dr. McFarland of that Institution made a strong case for the benefits of physical and occupational therapy in the treatment of PSP. It was advanced that physical therapy would be effective in preventing falls, and aiding general mobility and prevent the formation of contractures (abnormal muscle tightening and/or shortening). And, it was suggested that speech therapy would be valuable for addressing all forms of PSP induced speech problems. From my experience with having put Florence through all such "therapy", I submit that none of these assertions will provide any long term (over 6 months) benefit to a PSP patient. In fact, such suggestions create undue expectations for both the patient and the caregiver and can contribute to increased anxiety for both.

In retrospect, the year 2010 turned out to be a pivotal one. While home health care had provided frequent and excellent exercise training for Florence, by mid-2010 it was clear that inadequate physical improvement (if any at all) was occurring through therapy and adequate "progress" could no longer be shown. For Medicare to continue home health support, regular improvement in physical condition was needed. But, in reality, Florence's state was worsening, not improving, and falls were more frequent despite all therapeutic efforts. As a result and with the agreement of all parties concerned, the Home Health Care program was discontinued.

TERMINATION OF HOME HEALTH

We were now left with no assistance, agency or personal, making matters difficult for me. I feared leaving home over concern that Florence would fall in my absence. I could no longer rely on her promise to remain in bed while I was gone. But, there were times when I was left without a choice. Shopping was necessary as were my personal appointments for dentists, doctors, etc. And, things were becoming increasingly stressful as Florence lost her ability to manipulate the telephone and could no longer make or receive phone calls. That left her totally unable to communicate should something bad happen in my absence. Since I had no family available to help during the day, I sought to employ a medically experienced person. But, where to look? I finally contacted *Care.com*, an online agency which hosts health care position descriptions that may be responded to by interested persons. I listed a description for a part time position and received ten applicants via email within the first day. Several were interviewed, and one was selected to work three hours each Wednesday afternoon.

Florence's mobility and balance decline continued unabated. One morning she rose from the lift chair and walked across the living room toward the bannister for stairs leading to the second floor. Suddenly, with no warning, her head tilted back and she traced her steps backwards, rapidly, and out of control until she flopped into her lift chair. This happened so quickly that I did not have time even to rise from my chair and catch her. This occurred sporadically thereafter, especially the flopping into the chair (a typical PSP symptom) when attempting to sit down. A frightening prospect by itself, but we had earlier booked an Alaska cruise along with my sisters and their families for September of 2010. Moreover, since the ship was due to depart shortly, I had no choice but to cancel our trip. I couldn't imagine trying to prevent Florence's serious falls on a cruise ship when such incidents were nearly uncontrollable on dry land. This was of no matter to either the cruise line or the trip insurance company all of whom determined that my wife's inability to travel was the product of a preexisting condition. Thus, we lost both a substantial amount of money and the opportunity to see Alaska. It is important to know that trip cancellation insurance was also a wasted expense. Beware, if you have been treated for a condition prior to insurance enrollment. Should that condition prevent your travelling, trip insurance will not be of use.

All of our married lives, Florence and I shared a queen sized bed (never graduated to a king-sized one) and slept comfortably together therein. Circumstances were now causing this arrangement to be untenable. In her fits of anxiety, Florence constantly twisted and turned making sleep difficult for both of us. Incontinence grew to be a continual problem and a general low level of muscle pain added to her agitation. She constantly needed to change body positions in an attempt to be more comfortable. An adjustable bed would be helpful, but it was clear that what she truly needed was a hospital bed in a room of her own. In this way, she could continually adjust the bed at night without disturbing my sleep. She was no longer comfortable sitting in her lift chair for any length of time so a hospital bed would provide a useful alternative. Despite the potential benefits Florence was not sanguine about the notion. "I guess that my marriage is over," she complained in response **to** the new sleeping arrangements. I begged her not to feel that way, but I couldn't find another way to permit us both to find comfort as well as getting sufficient sleep. She was never one to argue for long so ultimately, a fully adjustable hospital bed was purchased and placed laterally against the wall within the guest bedroom. A half-length rail on the open side of the bed was installed to prevent her from falling out. Unfortunately, the bed rail was not as totally effective as originally anticipated because she did not simply tumble from normal movements during her sleep. She was also plagued with a condition of inner restlessness, called *akathisia,* which caused her to crawl out of bed, time after time, both day and night.

Falls also arose from self-toileting attempts or walking about by herself irrespective of the dangers. I had affixed handgrips to the bedroom, hallway, and bathroom walls through which she gained some measure of stability as she worked her way along. The bathroom was directly across the hall from the bedroom, and only a few steps were required to get there. Several large hand grips placed on shower walls lent stability during showers. I adjusted the bed to its lowest point to reduce the effects of a fall and placed a full length pad on the floor next to the bed. Even with such precautions, daily, at one time or another, I would hear the sound of a large thud she made when she fell. I bought a bicycle safety helmet and instructed her to put it on whenever she intended to walk around. The idea was to reduce head trauma from falls and it served that purpose several times. One morning I heard a resounding thud, much louder than usual. I rushed from my bedroom to find her flat on the hall floor crying after colliding head first with the hall drywall leaving a six inch hole in her wake. Of course, this time, she had failed to put on her helmet. A terrible fall indeed, and a concussion seemed inevitable even though she did not lose consciousness. I taught myself to tune my ears to any sound suggestive of a potential fall. When such a noise was detected, I would spontaneously rush to her room in hopes of catching her before she fell or at least to assess her condition. I came to hate that "falling sound" and tried other things to reduce its frequency. I purchased a full length, high safety rail so that falling or climbing out of bed would be much more difficult. While it was somewhat helpful, at times she would crawl over it anyway. Of course, she did it once too

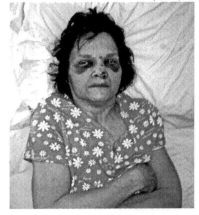

often and fell hard face down on the floor. As shown in this photograph, she suffered a swollen face, two black eyes, a broken nose, and two cracked ribs from that incident. Florence felt guilty and fearful after this fall; fearful that my patience was nearing an end. "Please don't leave me," she pleaded,

AFTER THE FALL

whereupon I did everything I could to convince her that I would always be with her as I had promised on our wedding day. Fewer falls ensued as she grew weaker. On some days we would simply hold hands and watch TV or listen to music. On pleasant days, I would wheel Florence out on our deck to absorb the sights, sounds and smells of nature. Florence still enjoyed good foods and to this point, we always ate dinner together. For variety, I routinely prepared a different requested dish for each meal. She enjoyed a wide range of dishes. Cod fish was a favorite as was barbequed steak, spaghetti, Shepherd's pie, king crab, soups, ham and chili, and these were always available in the freezer to accommodate her dinner urges. When dinner was ready, I would position her at the table in her wheelchair so that we might share the food together. Later, around the mid-point of her disease, I would cut up her food into small bits and feed it to her with a small spoon or fork (available on Amazon.com). However, as the disease progressed, this process grew increasingly difficult as her ability to open her mouth declined and she became less able to chew effectively.

4

Hospice Care

_____

HOSPICE IS A SERVICE

By September, 2010, Florence required considerable attention throughout the day and night. She needed comforting, food preparation and feeding along with toileting assistance (about every two hours), laundry, etc. The tasks were becoming just too great for me to accomplish alone on a daily basis. Someone mentioned that I should look into hospice care for assistance. I had heard of hospice in hospitals for cancer patients in particular, but other than that, I knew nothing about it. I decided to investigate to see whether hospice could offer us any benefits.

I soon discovered that "hospice" is a service, not a place, and it is provided in a hospital, skilled nursing facility, or a patient's home. It is available to persons of all ages even including children. Hospice care focuses on palliation of the terminally ill which means that all efforts are directed toward relieving physical and psychological pain and alleviating problems associated with a disease without dealing with the underlying cause.

The term *hospice* first came into use in the mid-1800's to describe the provision of care for dying patients. Through the efforts of British physician Dame Cicely Saunders, in the 1950's and 60's, organized hospice care in hospitals and nursing homes was begun. In the United States, hospice care started in 1974 with the opening of "Connecticut Hospice" in Branford by Florence Wald. Then, significantly, in 1978, a U.S. Department of Health, Education, and Welfare task force reported that:

> "The hospice movement as a concept for the care of 'the terminally ill and their families , is a viable concept and one which holds out a means of providing more humane care for Americans dying of terminal illness while possibly reducing costs. As such, it is the proper subject of federal support."

Following this recognition, hospice programs began to develop in earnest in the U.S., but legislation at that time was somewhat restrictive in that it provided for a maximum lifetime benefit of only 210 hospice days or about 7 months per patient. This limitation became widely known by the public and was misunderstood, even to this day. In reality, and of great significance, the 210 day lifetime limit per patient was eliminated and totally replaced with "unlimited care" language in 1990. This hospice benefit is now included under Medicare Part A. This is important because essentially all Americans aged 65 and older qualify for the benefit without necessarily having to enroll in Medicare Part B.

In September, 2010, I contacted several hospice companies to determine whether this form of assistance might be available to us. This proved to be a wise decision and was actually was a lifesaver for me. Up until then, I had thought that hospice care was only available for persons in the final months of their life but, with the 210 day limit having been eliminated, that concern was unfounded. To qualify for the program, a patient's primary care physician must first submit a form certifying that his/hers illness is terminal. Thereafter, enrollment is straight forward. There is an *evaluation of condition* process performed by a nurse practitioner every two months to renew hospice support from Medicare. In practice, people can receive benefits for several years if necessary.

Under hospice care, Medicare becomes the primary insurer. Any additional plan that one may carry, such as a Medicare Advantage insurance, offers no benefits while a patient is under hospice care. However, it is useful to continue separate insurance should a condition or circumstance arise outside the purview of the hospice program such as diagnosis or therapy of a different condition. A basic requirement of Medicare approved hospice care is that the patient receive palliative care only. In this way it is quite the opposite of the Medicare Home Therapy Program that we were enrolled in earlier. Again, should the need for some form of treatment classed as "therapy" arise, even, for example, when becoming a participant in a clinical trial for a new therapeutic drug, hospice care would most likely be suspended during this period and insurance coverage would need to revert to any secondary policy held.

Soon after Florence enrolled in hospice, we noted online that a promising new drug called *Davunetide* by Allon Therapeutics of Vancouver, B.C., Canada had received fast track approval from the U.S. Food and Drug Administration (FDA) for treatment of PSP in the United States. Allon showed that Davunetide reduced tau protein impairment in mice specially bred to replicate normal tau induced pathology. This and encouraging results from preliminary clinical trials in humans led to the proclamation by Allon that Davunetide was "…the most advanced tau therapy in the world." Needless to say, we were very excited when we saw this and held high hopes that a beneficial drug may finally be on the horizon. But, large scale clinical trials were required for FDA approval. In August of 2010, Allon Therapeutics announced a, "Study to Evaluate the Safety and Efficacy of Davunetide for the Treatment of Progressive Supranuclear Palsy" in ClinicalTrials.gov. Official title of the study was "A Phase 2/3, Randomized, Double-Blind, Placebo-Controlled, Study to Evaluate the Safety and Efficacy of Davunetide for the Treatment of Progressive Supranuclear Palsy."

Coordination of this clinical trial was to be handled by the renowned Memory and Aging Center at the University of California at San Francisco, Parnassus Campus and directed by Dr. Adam Boxer. After pre-qualification, participation in the clinical trial required a monthly visit to their clinic in San Francisco to administer the drug or placebo. At this point, no additional sites were yet established near where we lived. Travel was a difficult undertaking for Florence, but we would be willing to make the monthly excursion anyway if we felt it would be worthwhile. For us, the deciding factor was that this was a double blind clinical trial which meant that Florence would have a 50-50 chance of receiving a placebo rather than *Davunetide* throughout the trial, and that no financial support was available to assist with travel. On this basis we reluctantly decided against participating. We would have to wait for the outcome and hope that it would be successful enough for the drug to become widely available. But sadly, on December 18, 2012, Allon Therapeutics announced that the clinical trial to assess the potential of *Davunetide* for curing PSP had failed to show efficacy. As a result the company decided to terminate any additional research and would allocate no further capital to R&D to *Davunetide*. This announcement ended our hope for an effective medication, because no other truly promising drug is/was in the pipeline.

HOSPICE IN A NURSING HOME?

Around this time, I also explored the implications of long term hospice care in a skilled nursing facility (rather than at home) should my daily caregiving tasks eventually overwhelm me or should my health suddenly degenerate. I engaged an attorney specializing in elder care law who informed me of essentially the only government program available for long term care of the elderly. Nursing facility care is quite expensive, and all nursing homes I researched, even the poorest in terms of state ratings, bill at a minimal base rate of from $200/day or $6000/month and up. Of course, one must expect substantial additional charges for things like extra services, phone calls, T.V., etc. The only government supported programs for long term care is in the hands of the states through Medicaid (but not Medicare) for those people of limited income who are financially eligible. Programs vary from state to state, and some states provide financial assistance in either home or nursing home while others have a strict nursing home requirement. States also differ on the amount, duration, and breadth of services covered, rates of payment, and methods of administering the program. Thus, state Medicaid laws and procedures must be carefully examined in each case.

Spousal Impoverishment Laws allow the spouse remaining at home to protect a portion of income and resources when only one spouse needs nursing home care. Ostensibly, the objective of such laws is to prevent husband and wife from being reduced to abject poverty from nursing home costs. But, the procedures necessary to successfully fulfill requirements for Medicaid assistance are complex. There are innumerable pitfalls, so qualified legal aid along the way from an elder care lawyer would be most helpful if not absolutely necessary. Basically, the story goes something like this; if family income is below a defined threshold amount, there can be a division of assets and resources between the two spouses as determined by a local Social and Rehabilitation Services (SRS) office from all assets listed on a Resource Assessment and Allowance Determination form. Certain assets are not included (are protected from) asset division. These include the home and contents, one car, some personal possessions, and burial related assets. Home spouse may also keep income up to $1,650 per month. Not protected, however, are IRAs and other retirement programs which means that 50% of any such program immediately goes into the SRS hat, and should funds from any retirement program be taxable, federal and state income taxes would reduce net worth even further if cashed in immediately to fulfill spousal Medicaid obligations.

SELECTING A NURSING HOME

If a skilled nursing facility will be required for longer term care, it is prudent to first investigate local facilities. For example, there are about 25 nursing homes in Kansas City, Missouri plus a near equal number in surrounding towns all of which have been rated by the State of Missouri. Ratings for nursing homes in virtually all other states in the U.S. are also available and can be consulted on a single website, **Nursinghomerating.org**. This valuable site contains excellent information for each facility including: description, address, nursing home statistics such as number of beds and occupancy, overall and Individual ratings, inspection deficiencies, complaints, staffing information, and quality measures as determined by the Department of Health and Human Services. When such information is compared for one facility versus another, a dramatic range in quality will be found. Even so, the overall rating by itself will probably not be the only successful predictor in selecting a nursing home. When reviewing the ratings for the 25 Kansas City skilled nursing facilities, for example, I found the range in individual ratings to be from 1 out of 5 (the worst) to 5 out of 5 (best). Rating Frequencies were; #1 (2 facilities); #2 (13 facilities); #3 (5 facilities); #4 (3 facilities); #5 out of 5 (2 facilities). It would seem logical to choose the highest rated facility first, but limitations may be expected such as available bed space, whether or not Medicare and/or Medicaid is accepted, whether the facility will accept short term patients, e.g., under respite care, proximity of the facility, or whether a patient in a specific condition is acceptable. Thus, even after due diligence, there is no guarantee that a patient can be placed in a first choice, high quality facility. Sometimes, a patient might be "fortunate" (an oxymoron) to be accepted in any quality of nursing home.

HOSPICE SERVICES PROVIDED

Home hospice enrollment turned out to be a great benefit for us as it has been for multitudes of other people. To understand the service, it is good to know the legal obligations of a hospice company. Any Medicare Certified hospice company is charged to provide the following services.

1. Routine home care at the patient's residence, hospital or at a licensed skilled nursing facility.
2. All medications related to hospice diagnosis.
3. Supplies and medical equipment related to hospice diagnosis
4. Trained volunteer assistance
5. Respite care
6. Continuous round-the-clock care at near death period
7. Personalized bereavement support

Multiple hospice companies exist in most metropolitan areas of the United States. While each of them is theoretically required to provide the general services above, it is important to appreciate that individual companies differ greatly in the extent and quality of their performance for each criterion. Unfortunately, reliable ratings are less easy to find for hospice companies than for nursing homes and sub-par performance is difficult to identify. Ratings are based on consumer input rather than State evaluations. Management and sales personnel of all firms will most likely promise the best of care during initial presentations to potential customers. Still, in our experience, it is wise to judiciously review each hospice company for performance through discussions with several past and present patients and their families, and to review any public ratings that may exist. You will be surprised by the differences, and it is far preferable to put your loved one in the hands of the best local service than suffer frrom the frustration of the worst. Unfortunately for us, the first company I chose proved to be totally unsatisfactory over a period of six months. Staffing was too thin, often not on time for appointments, and highly changeable; management was largely unresponsive or hostile to any complaints or concerns, and only a modicum of supplies were provided, and then only grudgingly after repeated requests. After such experience, I did some further due-diligence and finally switched to a hospice with a far better record and a rare 5 star rating. This, the second one was great to deal with, performed all of the fundamental hospice duties in exemplary fashion, and regularly contributed even more than asked. Our experience for each of the service categories for the second hospice company is described below.

- <u>Routine home care at the patient's residence, hospital or at a licensed skilled nursing facility.</u> - A designated case registered nurse was assigned to visit the patient two times per week and generally oversees the program of care including medication ordering and pill inventory. She (or he) checks vital signs including blood pressure, temperature, blood oxygen level, heart rate, and listens to lung and abdomen sounds. A bath aide visits three or more times a week (whether at home or in a facility), as needed, to bathe or shower the patient. This service is extremely valuable to maintain hygiene and ward off bedsore development. As the disease worsens, showering requires increasing physical effort because of patient immobility. Commonly, the patient must be transported by wheelchair and is assisted while showering. In the home, the aide also routinely changed linens, kept a close eye out for bed sores or chaffing and informed the case nurse of any concerns. She also brushed Florence's teeth and tried to maintain oral care for her. This was important to avoid and dental related infections as Florence became unable to do so herself. In our experience, a good bath aide was an indispensable contributor to hospice care. In addition, a chaplain and a social worker each visited once or twice a month. The relevance of both became more apparent as the disease worsened. Valuable assistance was offered for such things a funeral arrangements, bereavement assistance, religious needs, nursing home arrangements, if desired, etc.

• <u>All medications related to hospice diagnosis.</u> This includes all prescribed drugs approved for the condition plus, depending upon the particular hospice provider, such expensive over-the-counter items as, *Miralax, Simply Thick*, Ibuprofen gel and tablets, *Mucinex* along with laxatives, and suppositories, plus body lotions, salves and creams designed to prevent or treat bed sores. It is worthy of note that hospice prescribed medications are not subject to the "Donut Hole" limitations of

Medicare Part D which would have been financially significant if Florence was not under hospice care.

• Supplies and medical equipment related to hospice diagnosis. Typical equipment provided on an as needed basis includes hospital bed, over the bed table, bedside commode, walkers, canes, wheelchair, shower chair, nebulizer machine for inhalation treatments with such solutions as *Ipratropium – Albuterol*, oxygen concentrator or portable oxygen tanks, and a trapeze over the bed. The trapeze was beneficial to Florence for a year or so to exercise her arms and help pull her out of bed. Its value declined after that as her ability to manipulate her hands and arms declined. Supplies included disposable underwear (like Depends), disposable chucks (which are waterproof bedding under-pads), massive numbers of disposable examination gloves and many other day to day items like powders and salves.

• Trained Volunteer Assistance. (Rarely available in my experience because of volunteer shortages in this area). In theory, volunteers would sit with the patient while the primary caregiver rests; is absent; or run errands; and would help with light homemaking chores. However, the volunteer is not allowed to conduct any form of medical aid or to supply medications to the patient and can only phone the hospice or the primary caregiver if something "medical" is needed.

• Respite Care. Provided for the patient in a hospital or skilled nursing facility for a period of up to 5 days every two to three months when the care provider needs a period of rest from duties. Support is not available if the patient remains at home.

In theory, this would seem to be a great benefit for a sole caregiver. In practice results may be altogether different, and it is indeed unfortunate that no form of respite time is allowed for the patient when at home. Success or failure (usefulness or not) of this benefit depends upon the type of illness, the condition of the patient and the quality of care offered by the individual nursing facility. No one in my family had ever spent time in or was familiar with a skilled nursing facility. Thus, I was totally naive with what goes on within once a patient is wheeled into a room. At the very least, I expected compassionate, attentive, and proper care of a loved one who was confined there in my absence. If only that were universally true! I experimented twice with two different nursing homes and wound up being completely dissatisfied. Despite having interviewed the administration of several different nursing homes, having been promised great things by all including very rapid reaction times to patient calls, and having chosen ones with the highest patient ratings, our results failed to turn out as promised. What follows are our experiences with the skilled nursing facilities we dealt with. What is written below is not intended to be a categorical diatribe inclusive of the entire nursing home industry, only pertinent to the ones we had experience with.

WHAT A DEAL @#@#

To prepare for my first respite period of five days, we toured the facilities of five nursing homes and met with the management of each. At our onsite meetings, we were guaranteed by all of prompt and compassionate care, but when we left, we were soon notified by four of the five facilities that Florence would not be accepted during my respite period. Puzzling result but at least one nursing home agreed to accept her.

When it came time for me to leave on a five day respite trip to Florida, to spend time with our daughter, I was apprehensive over Florence being alone, so her mother, at age 85, came to accompany her each day during my absence. A van from the facility transported both Florence and her mother, and upon arrival, both we were guided to a nicely appointed single room set aside for use only by respite care patients. I drove separately and tagged along to oversee. Furniture, including the hospital bed, was mahogany in color, there were two guest sofas, a wall mounted cable television, coffee and two end tables. Quite nice a facility indeed compared with any other that we had seen. Their idea, and it is a good one, is that comfortable surroundings would help dampen the negative effects of being away from home. Oh, if it were only that easy! Florence donned a new pajama set and I hung the remaining sets in the closet. I went over the entire medication schedule with the case nurse who guaranteed me that all pills would be given as ordered at the times stated. It was now dinner time and the three of us went down the hall to the cafeteria. Food was predictably poor in flavor, but it always is in such places, not unexpected. When we returned to the room we were shocked to find that all of the new pajama sets that I had hung up in the wardrobe were missing. And, new lingerie from the dresser drawers had been filched. I was furious, and was outspoken to members of management (few were around on Sunday when we arrived) of just how displeased I was. We went through the facility laundry to be certain that the clothing was not there by mistake. It was not. I was then promised that the missing articles would definitely be found and returned. It never, happened! Either there were outside thieves (unlikely) or workers hours were so mysterious that no one could discover who was on duty at the time of the theft. The next morning I left town for Florida and Florence's mother remained by her side. After I arrived in Florida, it didn't take long for my phone to ring. Medications were never supplied in time, often being as much as two hours late. Not a good thing given her condition and sensitivity to drugs. I complained to management, was promised that things would improve, but they never did. Nursing assistants and aides only infrequently entered the room, contrary to what we had been lead to believe. At night, Florence regularly thrashed about, kicked off sheets and blankets and often remained uncovered and chilled for up to four hours before anyone noticed. Forget the bedside call button. When depressed, a light would go on in the hall above the door, but it must not have been connected to any central point. No aide or nurse ever responded to it, and often they walked right past the door when the light was on. It did not seem unreasonable to me that someone was obliged to respond to the call button. Florence regularly needed pain medication, but not on a convenient schedule. Too bad! Her mother was livid through much of this, complained mightily, and brought prepared food from home so that Florence was able to eat on a regular schedule. I, of course, was given daily if not hourly reports. Some respite, huh! Florence lost five pounds of weight in five days. When I returned, I was not so politely informed that because we were so troublesome, we would no longer be welcome guests at that facility. Who would want to be? But their enmity was still surprising given the thievery and the difficult times Florence had experienced.

ONCE IS NOT ENOUGH!

Six months later, I decided to experiment with the respite concept once again, but decided to choose a different facility in hopes that Florence would receive better treatment. After several interviews and rejections we found what appeared to be a mutually agreeable facility. Ideally, I would certainly benefit from a period of relief from my caregiving chores every so often as prescribed in respite care. While visiting my daughter in Florida during the first period, my time on the beach was mainly devoted to sleep. It was nice not to be constantly on call (except for phone messages), but now, after the last nursing home experience, my level of confidence and trust was low indeed. So, this time, while I elected to try another facility, I was to remain close by to evaluate the goings on after Florence was admitted. Following a convincing sell job, including guarantees of near constant attention for Florence, no thievery, and a super-rapid response to call button alarms, I was confident of this nursing home even though it was a longer driving distance than the first one. Small inconvenience if the service was superior. Well, it was not. Same old – same old. Turned out that lack of call button response, unreliable medication delivery, lack of patient care, etc. were as unsatisfactory as in the prior institution. Never mind the promises. During the entire period, I never saw the same aide or nurse twice during my regular visits. Shifts were constantly changing with different personnel scheduled each time. And, good luck if you needed any form of special attention during meal time. Mid-week I stopped by the facility to visit Florence at noon. I went to her room and found her gone so I headed for the cafeteria. There she was, sitting alone at a large circular table with a tray of food before her. I was shocked, and felt so sad for her. Tears still well up in my eyes remembering the sight of such neglect. Skilled treatment, indeed! At this stage of her condition, she was unable to feed herself and nursing home administration was properly notified of this in advance. I confronted the first person with a badge I saw and asked what had happened to Florence's feeding. I was told that Florence wouldn't open her mouth wide enough for them to feed her with a standard fork or spoon so they moved along to patients who were more cooperative. Bastards! Even though Florence hated the food, I did manage to coax her into swallowing some of it after which I wheeled her back to her room. After this incident, my private-pay aide was rescheduled to be with Florence throughout each two hour dinner period to ensure that some essential nutrition was provided every day even if we needed to supply it from home ourselves. One day my private aide entered the room to find Florence lying on the floor. She had fallen out of bed and was not discovered by nursing home staff during the two hour period since she fell. Can you imagine this? In a hospital setting it is generally established that should a patient be on the floor, any period longer than 5 minutes is arithmetically deemed to significantly increase the odds of infection. What would one suppose the chances of infection would be after 2 **hours** on the floor? I protested vehemently about such lack of attention but too little avail. Administration at the facility stated that full length bed rails were not allowed to keep patients from falling out of bed because such a practice was considered to be RESTRAINT which is illegal under state law. And as well, administration argued that we should not expect nursing home staff to be everywhere at once. So, I guess that it is better to simply let patients fall, hurt themselves, and simply lay on the floor for hours, whether day or night, rather than be "Restrained." One can only imagine who dreamed up this hard and fast rule! What is more, since the facility did not even provide a television for her, I brought one from home so that she would have something to watch. But, for the entire 5 day period, cable was never connected to the television despite daily promises to me that it was to be hooked up immediately. From all of this, it was apparent that this, the second facility, offered no improvement over the former and, similarly, showed no obvious concern for its patients. At the end of the stay, as I wheeled Florence out to the car to return home, tears ran down her cheeks as she whimpered, "This place is just a prison for old women who come here to die." During her stay she had lost ten pounds and began to look frail. That was it! No matter how long it took, no matter how wearisome my caregiving would become, there would be no "respite periods" for me if it meant that Florence had to spend even one more day in a "skilled nursing facility" of the quality I had encountered. Given the very poor experiences in the two nursing homes that had already "treated" Florence, I still hoped to find other nursing facilities which were substantially better (a 5 rating for example) in their treatment of patients; but, "Don't count on it," I was told repeatedly, by members of my hospice team who also treat many people in local nursing homes. Then, of course, there is the matter of whether any suitable nursing home administration (if one exists) would even accept Florence. Eight of ten nursing homes visited, when I originally searched for a facility to perform respite care, turned Florence down because (they claimed) they were not prepared to care for someone in Florence's condition! What a sad commentary on senior health care! What happens to someone when no facility will accept the person for one reason or another and there is no one else to provide care? Certainly, there are fine facilities out there somewhere, but, sadly, I was not fortunate enough to encounter one.

• Continuous Care. To be provided by a registered hospice nurse in-the-home or institution on a round-the-clock basis when a patient's health status sharply declines to the point where death is imminent. This level of care is intended to replace the need for hospitalization at the end of a patient's life, and in our case, this offering turned out to accomplish just that. But be aware! Not all hospice companies offer 24 hour service even during final days which would make matters even more difficult and stressful at the time of death. It would be wise to seek guarantees of 24 hour care as necessary from any hospice one would subscribe with.

- <u>Personalized Bereavement Support</u>. Assistance during and after final days for at least one year. Major assistance with what to do "when your spouse dies." There is much more to handle than just funeral related matters including notification of death documents provided by the hospice so that a coroner need not be contacted by the family. Support groups are maintained to assist those who have lost a loved one. I did not avail myself of bereavement support groups early on because my strong family ties seemed to accomplish all that could be done. Things would change in time as waves of grief overcame me and I then reached out for assistance.

PROBLEMS WITH PAIN MANAGEMENT

By 2011, Florence's general pain level had gradually increased, and had created a major challenge for me to come up with tolerable pain killing medications. We made contact with experienced major institutions such as The Memory and Aging Center, UCSF to solicit suggestions beyond usual candidates such as ibuprofen, *Percoset*, and *Roxanol*. Nothing new was suggested. Since she was suffering muscle cramping and loss of fine motor control of arms and hands (dystonia) and pain, hospice people and I decided to try *Flexeril* (a muscle relaxant). What a mistake! A 5 mg tablet was administered at bed time in hopes of aiding sleep through reduced pain. Rather, and unbeknownst to me, she was very intolerant of the drug and soon began to hallucinate. I had fallen asleep, but heard thumping and awoke to find her walking down the hall talking to who she thought was our daughter. What a shock! First, she had not been able to walk that normally in years, and secondly, I had never seen her to be so mentally out of control. I had great difficulty in convincing her to return to bed, and I sat with her for the rest of night to prevent another walking occurrence. Thank goodness that she had not gone in the other direction and fallen down the stairs. All night and into the next day she continued to hallucinate, spiders were seen on the ceiling, the walls and the bed, colors in the room kept changing, other imaginary creatures occasionally passed by, and discussion continued with nonexistent people. This was just another example of her unpredictable response to a drug and throughout her illness, great caution was needed during the introduction or removal of any drug.

LOSS OF MOBILITY

Early in 2011, Florence was far too unsteady to walk unaided, and whenever she tried, she fell. She could stand up with minor assistance, but was too unsteady to move about without assistance. This meant that human presence was absolutely required for all toilet trips which were quite frequent through the day and night. While time consuming at home, lack of mobility also rendered any lengthy trip by automobile impossible unless another woman was along to assist. While I could help Florence to the toilet door, obviously I could not enter the female toilet in a public location. And, the same was true for airports should we be flying.

By this time, her leg muscles were atrophying, particularly her thighs. She had become a thin person of five feet three inches and just over 105 pounds. Muscles in her hands were tightening and fingers assumed a gnarled state making it difficult for her to grasp anything. Her hands had also become sensitive to any form of contact and were painful when touched. From then on, there could be no hand holding between us. Simultaneously, her eyesight was weakening and several sets of reading glasses with different magnifications were tested. A few offered a modicum of benefit, but for only a brief time. Hearing and cognition, thus far, seemed to be relatively steady. Meanwhile, her underlying pain level was becoming an even greater problem, especially shoulders, arms and hands. *Percoset* was helpful but inadequate, morphine sulfate solution (*Roxonal*) given orally was largely ineffective, but a 20% ibuprofen gel (salve) applied to arms and hands did reduce pain. We tested the anti-inflammatory drug *Mobic* (*Meloxicam*) and quickly found that it was helpful in reducing her general or overall pain level (from a level of 3 to a level of 1) and remained effective over a period of several months. But as expected, efficacy ultimately became less with time.

I continually placed great emphasis on her nutrition. Since the second and last nursing home episode, Florence was underweight and I tried to supply enough food (calories) for her three times a day in hopes of achieving weight gain. This included large quantities of meat dishes, high calorie smoothies, protein supplements, fruits, and the like. But the diet failed to have the desired effect and although she did not lose any more weight through this period, neither did she gain any.

CONTINUING MEDICATION CHALLENGES

Florence seemed to hold up fairly well, mentally, through all of this physical degradation, but now, she was showing signs of emotional weakening. I would sit with her while watching TV (she especially enjoyed the sensitivity of "The Waltons" and the children of "Little House on the Prairie"). Small tears would often squeeze from the corners of her eyes as she remembered earlier days with her own family. She rarely complained about her circumstance (except when in pain), but every so often she would tell me, "I would give anything to be out of this body." Then one afternoon as I walked past her room I saw that she was fiddling with a bottle of pills. I went in and asked what was going on. "I am going to take all (30) of these *Percoset* pills," she replied.

"Can't let you do it," I stated as I took the bottle away. "What would become of me if you swallowed all of these pills? I would be crushed and alone without you."

Once again she said, "I want out of this body!"

The subject of medication was a continuing palliative challenge throughout this malady, and actually became a regular topic unto itself. Incidentally, it is important that mention of any drugs throughout this book is in no way an endorsement of them nor a recommendation for their adoption to any other person's circumstance. Each instance elaborated here is specific to Florence and relates only to how we cared for her as we went along. It was not done willy-nilly! After suggestion, each prescription was carefully considered by the primary physician along with the hospice registered nurse assigned to oversee the case. There was little to go on from the literature and since no curative drugs were available, all that could be done was to take a stab (with drugs) at symptoms as they appeared. There were successes and failures, and once a drug was begun, there was the threat of unpredictable secondary effects when the drug was discontinued. Zoloft in particular is one which is difficult to wean a person from. The same was true for Carbo/Levo which by 2011 provided no obvious benefit except that Florence was anxious without it. But, I needed to also supply *Risperidone* at bedtime to offset enough Carbo/Levo induced anxiety to allow sleep. An obvious question here would be, "Why not just drop the bedtime Carbo/Levo?" That was attempted many times, but when this drug was eliminated at bed time, her mobility declined and she could not adjust blankets, position, etc., and in the morning she would often complain of being "frozen" meaning that she was almost totally unable to move. Liquid *Trazadone* was also supplied at bedtime as a sleep aide and it seemed to be regularly effective.

Soon after the onset of urinary incontinence, Florence suffered from frequent bouts of serious urinary tract infections (UTIs). Round and round we went at monthly intervals. First symptoms appeared then a prescription for the antibiotic *Ciprofloxacin* (Cipro) was provided for 5 days to knock the infection down. Urine was checked daily with test strips and samples were cultured when infection was indicated. Finally, an urologist we knew suggested use of the antibiotic *Bactrim* (sulfamethoxazole and trimethoprim) on a daily basis as a prophylactic. This idea was not accepted out of hand. Rather, there was some concern on the part of the primary care physician about the possible emergence of antibiotic resistant bacterial strains developing from continued use of *Bactrim*. While this prospect did exist, a similar risk occurred from repeatedly treating UTIs with *Cipro* to fight off recurring infections. The question then was which risk was greater. One which of itself like Bactrim can be quite harmful. Alternatively, Cipro is very effective in eliminating an infection once it is identified. In Florence's case, reinfections were very common so we decided to go ahead with *Bactrim*. Success! After following the *Bactrim* directive, urinary tract problems disappeared.

HOSPICE & OTHER AIDES

Not to be repetitive, but, I cannot truthfully describe caregiving at home without mentioning at some length the continued invaluable contributions of the hospice team assigned to Florence's care. There was Jodie, a forty year old bath aide who came 5 days a week to cleanse, shower, and comfort her. She and Florence grew close and she was thought of as a close friend. Each day during the week Florence looked forward to her arrival and would muster her best try at a smile when she came into the room. Jodie also sat with Florence for a time, changed linens as needed, and with no requests from me, went about the house emptying trash bins, and even changed my bed. All of this behavior was unique to Jodie (we had fill-in aides in Jodie's days off for comparison) and I couldn't imagine getting along without her. There were also others including the case nurse who checked vital signs, and patient condition two times a week, assisted with breathing problems and, kept a close tab on any potential aspirational pneumonia. In fact, I also looked forward to their coming so that I had someone to visit with. Sitting at home alone day after day with no outside human interaction did get a bit depressing.

Around this time, someone informed me that the county of my residence offered a "Senior Assistance Fund" to bolster the home caregiving of disabled seniors. I filed an application and was ultimately granted the assistance of an aide for a total of eight hours each week with time blocks being divided according to my request. I chose a two hour block (5-7 pm) each Tuesday through Friday. The program was administered through any one of several local home health care companies who would provide paid personnel. Usually these aides assisted in meal preparation and feeding, and on warm, sunny days they would load Florence into her wheelchair, put on her dark sunglasses and hat, and for a short while, roll her out onto the deck at the rear of the house. A nice diversion from the hospital bed. We experimented with a Geri Chair which is a multi-position reclining chair on wheels with head supports, elevated foot rests and over-the-lap tray. In theory, this should provide a comfortable alternative to a wheel chair when Florence was out of bed, but in reality the chair was not as useful as we had thought. Florence did not like sitting in it and the chair was so heavy and unwieldy as to be a major inconvenience. So my caregiving team was nearly assembled and I sought to complete it with the private hiring of a CNA (Certified Nursing Assistant) through *Care.com* to serve during the day on Saturdays and/or Sundays. This proved be a continuing challenge. I needed to have someone who was qualified to care for Florence during my absence and to perform light housekeeping duties while Florence slept. While I regularly hired some qualified people who became fond of Florence and did a good job of caring for her, after a few days, weeks, or months they would depart for one reason or another and I would need to resume the search for a replacement. I had to maintain a pool of two or three aides at a time to be confident that anyone would show up. This problem was constant and remained a major impediment to comfortable care. Florence was forced to respond to new aides constantly, and while she responded pretty well, it was nonetheless difficult for her. Of course, along the way I was also was fooled into hiring some untrained, not-so-good people who had serious personality problems, and seemed to enjoy making our lives difficult. They ultimately were soon dismissed amidst bizarre accusations of unfair treatment on our part etc. In an attempt to standardize care during weekend days, one excellent aide, Jennifer, wrote the following manifesto. It served as a guideline for new helpers as they came in to replace departing ones, and saved me from having to go through standard required caregiving duties repeatedly.

Weekend Duties and Tips for Caring for Florence

Please keep in mind that Florence is a grown woman who is aware of her surroundings and understands perfectly what you ask her, she is capable of deciding what she wants to eat at meal time, and will answer any questions you ask her to the best of her ability, at times she is hard to understand and may need to repeat herself, just be patient. I would suggest doing a little research on Supra Nuclear Palsy, in order to understand what is affected by this disease, as it may be of help to you.

Upon arrival, if Florence hasn't been toileted, take her to the bathroom, she may need fresh clothes. While in the bathroom make sure her bed is clean and dry, if a change is needed, you will find sheets and pads in the closet in her room. Grab a plastic bag from the bathroom cabinet for her used briefs, wipes and gloves, this will be tied up and discarded before you leave. Make sure to wash Florence's face in the morning, a warm washcloth will do fine. When she is done on the toilet, make sure to wash her peri-area, there are wipes as well as peri-wash in a spray bottle on the counter in the bathroom. I prefer to use wipes first, then a warm washcloth with peri-wash on it to finish up and ensure cleanliness. I usually offer to assist with brushing Florence's teeth before leaving the bathroom, she may need help brushing and have difficulty opening her mouth, do the best you can, she is able to rinse and spit just fine in the emesis basin that her toothbrush is kept in.

After assisting Florence back to bed you can decide what she would like for breakfast, she usually eats around 11:00. She can no longer open her mouth well so for breakfast you puree the following: 4 poached eggs, splash of flavored coffee creamer, 1 cup whey protein plus 1 Tbsp cocoanut oil, 2 fish oil tablets, 1 capful Miralax and 2 Tbsp 4% fat cottage cheese. Feed with 50 cc syringe. We usually also fix a fruit smoothie around 3 pm as well. Blend some yogurt and fresh fruit, add 2/3 of a scoop of protein powder, and blend well. Dinner is around 5:00 & most everything will be blended, you may have to use your imagination when making smoothies and blending meats, soups, etc. For example, with a can of ravioli, you will want to put some tomato soup in to thin it out for easy use of the 50 cc syringe. Remember, when using the syringes to dip the plunger into the oil, this will make it much easier to use.

Medicine should be given at 11:00 am, and again at 3:00 pm, see med list on the wall, next to the clock. Check with Mr. Shepard before giving Bisacodyl, as she hasn't been taking it daily. To keep busy, feel free to straighten Florence's room. If the dishes in the dishwasher are clean, I put them away and then put dishes in the dishwasher as we use them, if they need to be washed, I run it and then put them away. I wipe down counters, as well. Check to see if there is any laundry to be done, either to wash, or sometimes some has been started and will need to be finished, folded and put away. I just do what I can to help out, if I see something that needs done, I do it.

Jennifer

5

Phase III

_____

FEAR OF LONELINESS

As I reflected back upon expectations for my senior years, I not once anticipated that I would be the one providing long term care for my spouse. Indeed, I always expected the opposite from family history starting with visits with my bedridden paternal grandfather when I was a child. In his elder years, he suffered a series of strokes which left him dependent upon my grandmother's full time attention. Father would take me, his only son, with him to visit Grandpa at his home each Sunday morning. It was never a fun time for me since I rarely spoke with grandfather other than a quick hello and, instead, waited quietly while my father interacted with his parents and two sisters. A generation later, the stroke scenario was repeated when my father reached the age of 63 and when his brother was 65 years old, both became terminal stroke victims. This trait was so common on my father's side of the family that I fully expected the same outcome for me. I routinely warned Florence what she was likely to face in my senior years, and she accepted this with little obvious concern. Perhaps my mother's genetic contribution would protect me from that medical predisposition. I also never expected that I would be devoted enough to my lifelong partner to sacrifice all else in life solely for the sake of her long term care. Now, the youngest grandchildren's remembrances of Florence will only be a distant recollection of her in a sickened condition akin to that of me and my grandfather. That will be most unfortunate for them since they will miss out on all of the goodness, caring and love she would have given.

Days were growing very long for me with a seemingly endless list of duties sometimes even overtaxing my caregiving ability. Housekeeping, lawn care, grocery shopping, supply management, bill paying, etc. all had to be folded in. For a time, I began to feel quite sorry for myself. Often, I lacked the enthusiasm to even rise from bed and start the day; that is if I was aware of what day of the week it was. I needed a guidepost, like "Tuesday is trash day", or, in winter, "KU plays basketball on Wednesday nights" to keep focused. We were now in an age when over half of all marriages ended in divorce, when men and women preferred transitory live-in relationships over marriage, when my son's wife simply grew tired of him and their three children and left in favor of a new guy. But, despite such societal upheaval, here I was, an anachronism, still in love with my wife, despite all of her medical problems, and denying all others for as long as I could keep her alive. For a time, the specter of being alone for the remainder of my life constantly played on my mind and depression threatened to settle in. During most of our life, any free time was spent together, but now, there was no one to spend time with except at bedside. I missed being with the Florence I once knew, terribly. Enjoying trips together to the Ritz Hotel in Paris, cruising up the Amazon River, kicking up sand on the beaches of Bora Bora and Siesta Key, Florida, sharing fine dinners together at the Country Club Plaza in Kansas City, etc. Now, when I went shopping, I was always alone, and I would see couples walking hand in hand, enjoying one others company as Florence and I did for so many years. At other times, I would stop in at a local cafe and observe couples joyfully interacting, and making plans for the weekend. I was happy for these people, but at the same time I was sad for me. I doubted that I would ever enjoy this form of companionship again. It is a very difficult challenge to remain upbeat when at the same time life is ebbing away from your life-long partner. Such thinking was very depressing and counter-productive so I tried not to allow myself to fall victim to it for any significant period of time. In 2013, I turned 72 years of age and needed occasional medical attention of my own, aorta aneurysm surgery for example. Never a convenient situation because, when I was absent, I needed to find a qualified person to look after Florence until I returned. During especially serious times, one of my sisters would come to help, but this was not a constant solution. Sometimes a certified nursing assistant was hired full time to fill in for me. I worried at some length about what would happen to Florence if I became totally incapacitated. Full time assistance at home on a 24 hour basis would be cost prohibitive. Furthermore, since she was unable to open her mouth and could not chew normally, she would not be accepted into any nursing home unless she agreed to a gastrostomy (feeding tube directly into the stomach). The problem was that Florence was very much against this as spelled out in her Medical Directives. And, if I were to fall or otherwise become suddenly disabled, there would be no one here to call for help unless I signed up for Life-Alert which I didn't do.

NOW YOU SEE IT – NOW YOU DON'T

As the years of Florence's illness trudged past, I slowly adjusted to doing things alone and generally grew used to getting along without human interaction except chatter with aides during regular periods of hospice caregiving. Actually, the coming and going of aides whether hospice, home health or private pay somewhat softened the loneliness. I grew to look forward to their arrival just to be able to interact with someone; that is, until items began disappearing from my home. At first, favorite porcelain collectibles showed up missing from the china cabinet. I had complete trust in all of the ladies that came to my home to provide care for Florence, and I had absolutely no idea who the culprit(s) might be. Then, matters grew worse as prescription pain drugs began to disappear. *Percoset* was the prime target and since this was supplied by the hospice on a regular basis and, the agency was none too happy about such thievery. Much damage can be done to relationships when a thief is present among a supposedly caring staff. At first, and in the absence of any clues, all aides were suspect. The hospice had only one person on premises during the week on a daily basis, the bath aide. To be certain that she was not responsible, hospice management removed her from duty here and replaced her with a number of substitutes. Thefts continued! In fact, actions were even more devious. The project nurse and I placed all Percoset pills in a lock box and only she and I had keys. According to protocol, the nurse counted all remaining Percoset pills every Tuesday and Thursday. Lo and behold, pills disappeared at the same rate, irrespective of the supposed security of a lock box. What the hell! Did we have a professional thief on our hands under the guise of a nursing assistant? It is mystery that we never solved. Since we had no video evidence of the culprit, and could not prove our suspicions, we were left with only two possible candidates. Perhaps one was guilty perhaps both! I wish that then we had the inexpensive recording devices that are common today to help identify the culprit(s).

Then one day, Florence whispered to me, "I want to tell you something." I placed my ear next to her mouth as she struggled to whisper, "Mandy stole my rosary." On the wall next to her bed once hung a beautiful rosary with *Swarovski* crystal beads and a 24 k gold cross. "Are you sure," I asked. She nodded and stammered that Mandy thought that she was asleep and reached over her to lift the rosary. Mandy was a part time private-pay aide who had been with us for a few months. She was a 20 year old CNA (certified nursing assistant) who worked during the early part of each day at a nearby nursing home and then would spend a couple of hours in the afternoon with Florence three days a week. Although she was an attractive, pleasant person, she continually suffered from a broad range of personal problems stemming from a poor upbringing, and less than ideal living arrangements. By the time Florence told me about the rosary being missing, Mandy had left for the day so I phoned her to discuss issue. She emphatically denied theft of the rosary claiming that she would never do such a thing. Having personally observed the rosary hanging from the wall just prior to Mandy's arrival and noticed it's absence afterwards, I believed Florence, and did not accept the Mandy's denial. I instructed Mandy to return the rosary whereupon she repeated that she had not taken it. After this phone call, I saw neither the rosary nor Mandy again and she would no longer accept my phone calls. Unfortunately, that was not the end of all thievery. I had collected coins in a large bottle for several years, and the accumulation had grown to over $200.00. One day, after Mandy had left my employ, the change jar had been nearly emptied in a nefarious act by another of my aides. Generously, the thief left about $30.00 worth of change, thinking, I guess that I would not notice. Then suddenly, the only remaining box we had of *Fentanyl* transdermal patches disappeared. Florence only needed that strong of an anti-pain treatment once in a while. Since these patches were not continually used, it was impossible to pinpoint exactly when they were taken. So, I concluded that I had been the victim of two thieves rather than one. Quick review of which aide had been on duty at the time of the disappearance pointed directly to a home health aide that had been here for nearly a year. Very disappointing given all else I had to deal with, but I immediately replaced both the aide and the agency of her employ with another. Since then, I suffered no further thefts.

Caution should be exercised when connecting with a "Home Health Care" company. Many such franchised businesses are around and it is very difficult to gather independent information about the quality of one versus another. Management of each will provide an idealized answer to any question you might pose, but how do you find out about the experience of their aides who actually perform the home health care duties? What about background checks? And, will you be billed accurately and fairly. If a deposit is required up front, will they refund it if you transfer to another company? In my experience, the answer to these questions may well be "no," even when negative things (such as theft) happen. Never mind listening to promises of doing better, etc. which are routinely offered after mistakes. Look at the fine print in your contract and you will find a hidden clause which states that cancellation of services for any reason (including death of the patient) must be notified to the company at a minimum of 2 weeks prior to cessation of services or the deposit will not be refunded. This limitation happened to us and our deposit was confiscated when Florence died unexpectedly.

These experiences were most likely not unique to us, suggesting that great caution and oversight be must undertaken when allowing aides or other strangers into a patients home. Small recording devices would be quite a deterrent to thievery.

Hospice aides were of great help in the caregiving process as were most home health aides, but they could only be with Florence for a short time in any given day. Nighttime toileting sessions were frequent, often unpleasant, and were my obligation. For those who have not had to perform this task on a regular basis, it is very much like dealing with the soiled diapers of an infant on an adult scale during sleepy hours of the night. Sometimes I needed to go outdoors for a breath of fresh air during the process. I will always remember Florence's rejoinder during a particularly unpleasant toileting episode when I asked, "Where in our wedding vows did it say that I must do this." She quickly answered with one word, "Worse" as in ".. for better or for worse." I was appreciative that my hospice and other home health aides always took this job in stride during daytime hours. I don't know how they do it.

WHAT IF?

Once Florence was no longer ambulatory, and, hence, had become bedridden, my sisters and I contributed everything we could think of in the way of entertainment to reduce her daily boredom and discouragement. Together, we installed a television for her to watch and early on she could select channels including Netflix and Pandora with a remote. One sister supplied a DVD player and sent many DVDs. I bought an iPod with headphones and downloaded many of her favorite tunes. Also downloaded several audiobooks to her iPod including *Pride and Prejudice* and for a time she truly enjoyed listening to each of them. These steps did provide some measure of distraction and, hopefully, enjoyment for her, but as time passed she became unable to operate the remote control(s). When that point was reached, I needed to visit her room often during the day and evening to help her select movies, shows or songs, etc.

Theoretically, there should always be a professional facility option available as a backup to care for Florence or other people in a similar situation who prefer or are forced to accept institutionalization over home care. But, this option assumes that some licensed healthcare facility would accept her. None (to my knowledge) will administer food exclusively with a syringe even though this came to be the only effective feeding procedure for her at home. It is feared by many professionals that syringe feeding greatly increases the odds of inducing aspirational pneumonia. While this might be true in certain circumstances, we cannot see where this method was directly responsible for any abnormal problem here and to make certain, Florence's lung condition was monitored at least twice weekly by her hospice nurse, Leigh. If for some reason, Florence had to be admitted to a nursing home, a feeding tube would have to be inserted before they would accept her and Florence was dead against this procedure. Beside, after our experience earlier with two different nursing homes, I simply could not subject Florence to that style of life for as long as I was physically able to care for her. So here we were, innovating as we went along, certain of her future but not of the timing, feeling constant sadness and forgetting how to smile.

POWERS OF ATTORNEY

That brings us to the subject of *Durable Power of Attorney for Health Care and Health Care Directive*. This document authorizes someone (an agent) to make decisions on their behalf when too ill to speak for one's self along with specific instructions (the *Health Care Directive*), that specify what actions should be taken for their health when one becomes persistently unconscious or there is no reasonable expectation of recovery, e.g., tube feeding, dialysis, CPR and respirator. A power of attorney (POA) is made "durable" when a clause states that the document is to stay in effect for the duration of the medical incapacitation or disability. The durability provision, in effect, avoids the need to have a court appoint a guardian conservator. Always keep in mind that POA forms must be signed by the patient and witnessed by two people. This document stays in effect until it is revoked or until the signer's death and can only be revoked by the signer. This is an important document for a disabled person to file. Copies are provided to the Agent, The Primary Care Physician, and usually the sick person's attorney. This is often accompanied by a *Durable Financial Power of Attorney* that gives an agent the authority to handle simple or complex financial transactions. It is recommended that both documents be done separately but at the same time before the patient becomes too disabled to physically sign the documents. Should the patient be unable to sign, a court order will be required to complete the documents. A third document, *"Outside the Hospital DNR Request Form"* is also commonly prepared by seriously ill persons to limit the scope of emergency medical care. The Do Not Resuscitate (DNR) order here means that if the patient's heart stops beating or if breathing has stopped, no medical procedure may be used to restart breathing or heart function. This form is regularly required by health care facilities.

FURTHER DECLINE

By January 2012, Florence's condition was demonstrably worse than before and adjustments were needed in many phases of her care. She now was totally unable to get out of bed on her own, so at least falls from that source were eliminated. But, she could partially rise and stand when assisted and was able sit down in the wheelchair and on the commode with the help of an aide. Earlier I had set up walkie-talkies so that she could contact me for assistance if I was in a different room of the house, in the backyard, or simply waiting for her to finish in the bathroom. This worked out well for nearly a year, during which I was comfortable knowing that I was not out of contact with her at any time I was out of earshot. But, as time wore on, her ability to grip handholds, grippers, etc. declined and even walkie-talkies became redundant. She was not able to depress the send button or even hold onto the unit. The same had been true for the telephone for some time where she could not answer, hold or dial the phone and if I held it for her, she was very difficult to understand. As another approach toward communication, I set up a plug-in doorbell which rang just outside of her bedroom when she depressed a small call button to needed help. Not as good as the walkie-talkie, but it was effective until most fingers of each hand became fixed in a semi-curled position and thus, immobile. Muscles had contracted in her arms, hands and fingers and eventually became nearly rigid. By then the call button–doorbell combo was no longer helpful, and joined the lengthy list of redundant aids. Physical items that were once helpful like the bicycle helmet, canes, walkers and any other mobility related items were now also redundant. She could no longer reach or grip the trapeze to exercise her arms. Her thighs had shrunk to the diameter of my forearm. Contracted arm and hand muscles caused her near-constant pain that could not be effectively controlled by regular or opiate pain killers. Through experimentation, we found that application of topical 20% ibuprofen salve two of three times daily to arms and hands partially controlled the pain. Little else seemed to work.

FEEDING AND MEDICATION

Feeding was becoming difficult and took quite a long while as she suffered a much reduced capacity to open her jaws (mouth). It wasn't that her jaws were locked, permanently frozen, or otherwise mechanically compromised, she had simply lost most of her ability to control the opening and closing at will. And, the specter of aspiration was ever present.

Florence had always favored a blueberry pancake - bacon breakfast topped off with a bottle of *Boost* or *Ensure* for supplemental nutrition. That was changing. The only way for her to consume solid foods was to insert through the gap left in her teeth by the absence of the partial plate if her mouth was partially opened. How ironic! The gap in her teeth that almost certainly led to her current condition was the only portion of her jaw that would accommodate specialty feeding utensils like the tiny forks and spoons we purchased on the internet. Great care was required when giving her liquids through straws or by sipping since aspiration was now more common. If the drink consistency was not thick enough, choking would begin immediately no matter what the circumstance even if just taking a small pill. All liquids needed to be of high viscosity, at least equivalent to "honey", either on their own or when supplemented. In our experience, *Simply Thick* was the best commercially available thickening agent. It came as a gel, not a powder, was virtually tasteless, and was easily dispensed with the pump supplied with large bottles. Generally, depressing the pump handle once supplied about 0.5 ounce of gel. Her daily medication at this time consisted of a carbidopa-levodopa, 25-100 mg tablet (not the slow release type) at 4 hour intervals from 7 am until 11 pm. In addition, she received one *Zoloft* tablet, plus one *Mobic*, one *Mucinex* to loosen the ever present congestion, and one *Bactrim* tablet daily. *Atavan* liquid (1 ml of 2 mg/ml) was administered at bed time as was *Trazadone* and *Risperidone*, all aimed at helping her sleep. I wish to say once again that this regimen is not recommended for anyone else; it is just the one that I and my hospice team found to be effective for Florence. Clearly, after this long period of time, some of the drugs, i.e. carbo/levo, probably had become ineffective. But, if nothing else, it offered a placebo effect that I dared not to withdraw.

When first affected by PSP, Florence's face became near expressionless or masked and that condition persisted to one degree or another throughout. But by 2012, her face was subject to all manners of expression except a smile. Seemingly, her condition blocked this one form of communication. She would frown when disapproving, grimace in various contorted ways when in pain, and would cloud up facially with streaming tears when she felt upset. By mid 2012, her voice had weakened to the point where she could barely be heard unless a person's ear was placed next to her mouth. She regularly would lay in bed looking straight toward the ceiling unless uneasy or in pain whereby she would constantly twist and turn. Her bed was usually set at a 20% angle or greater to reduce aspiration and help her swallow the constantly accumulating phlegm. Throughout this, her cognition remained good and she could remember things from the past as well as peoples' names better than I.

By this time, constant toileting demands involving bladder and bowel incontinence was overwhelming. It seemed that trips to the bathroom went on non-stop day and night and I as well as my aides were developing back aches. To improve matters, we tried to reduce the bowel incontinence frequency. Attempts were made to improve regularity by adding both *Miralax* and fiber to her breakfast cocktail daily.

After a time we found that by doing so, she would request BM assistance within a slightly more predictable time frame.

FEEDING ADJUSTMENTS

Feeding had become an issue by mid-2012. Florence could no longer open her mouth sufficiently to eat solid foods at all, and I did not think that I could supply enough nutrition with a simple liquid diet of *Boost, Ensure* or equivalent. So for breakfast/lunch served each day at 11 am I developed the following combination which was pureed in a 26 ounce *Nutribullet* blender jar and fed with a 60cc irrigation syringe through the gap in her teeth. Ingredients were 3 ounces (6 pumps) of simply thick, 1 scoop (42 grams) of Body Fortress Super Advanced Whey Protein, strawberry flavor; 1 heaping teaspoon Equate Fiber Therapy Psyllium Husk Fiber; 4 lightly poached eggs, handful of frozen whole strawberries, B-complex vitamins plus a B_{12} tablet, 1 tablet broad spectrum vitamins, 1000 mg Vitamin D_3, 1 cap *Miralax,* 3 heaping tablespoons of 4% large curd cottage cheese, and finally, one tablespoon each of raw honey, extra virgin coconut oil, and strawberry flavored syrup. In our experience, this mixture was both flavorful and highly nutritious. Through its consumption, Florence at least maintained her weight at the level from the last nursing home lost. A small protein enriched smoothie was prepared each afternoon to take with the 3 pm carbo/levo pill. Dinner was a different matter. This was the meal at which she could make a decision between which meat dish she would like. Choices usually ranged from a number of frozen entrees by several suppliers like *Banquet* to home-made favorites like candied ham and she would decide what sounded good to her each day. Hopefully, I had anticipated her choice and had it available or had frozen it after a recent shopping trip. If not, I would immediately head for the grocery store. I considered it vital to satisfy her desires for the evening meal irrespective of any inconvenience. This gave her something to look forward to and to some extent enriched her life. What else did she have to brighten her day? Florence was especially fond of sweet and sour chicken if it was properly prepared. In earlier time, she was a master in the preparation of sweet and sour pork ribs following a recipe given to us by an old college friend named Jerry. She preferred the flavor of this dish (albeit now made with chicken) so often that I began preparing large batches and then freezing dinner sized portions for later use. Of course this, like all other dishes, had to be pureed before serving. Naturally, the original food texture was lost, and I was surprised that Florence continued to accept it. When using commercial sources like *Banquet* I would puree it with a chicken stock or pineapple juice diluent to achieve the right consistency. Particular care was required to avoid much in the way of spiced dishes. Even light spicing with red peppers caused her to choke and aspirate and had to be discarded. Now, if I could only think of something for me to eat.

I usually maintained a well-stocked freezer to accommodate any spur of the moment food desire that might come up at the end of the day. Often this stocking was influenced by weekly specials at the supermarket, and I may or may not ever create a dish from such bargains. While early in a day I may be enthusiastic about preparing a time consuming dish, but, later in the day, enthusiasm often ebbed in favor of something quick and/or easy if I was alone. It is indeed difficult (in my experience) to enjoy the process of meal preparation for ones-self when several hours were required.

NO REMISSIONS

Earlier I made mention of the fact that remissions are not to be expected for PSP, but like most maladies, there were "good days and bad days." resembling mini-remissions as the disease progressed. Sometimes, her condition would decline day after day for up to a couple of weeks to the extent that the process of rapid decline of itself seemed constant during these times. For example, when she first began to lose her voice, her speaking ability initially declined over a period of four weeks until she could no longer speak at all and along with it, her general responsiveness was greatly reduced. She would sleep or doze much of each day and would only wake during breakfast/lunch and dinner feeding times. But, after a level period of about a week, she regained the ability to at least whisper again and after a few more days, she might even pronounce a few words. Periods of rapid decline were very stressful for all of us caregivers because we had no idea when or if the decline would stop, or at least plateau. In the midst of such phases, we became less optimistic about her longevity. This was particularly true when she was suffering a decline in her ability to swallow which was generally accompanied by coughing and choking from aspiration. During a period like this, we became very worried that she soon might be unable to swallow all together and were uncertain how to deal with that eventuality. But, thank goodness, like the "Energizer Bunny", she would bounce back to near the starting point of the decline although not quite all the way back. That was true for many symptom classes. Each "bounce back" was encouraging, but as already mentioned, it was never all of the way or long lasting.

It is difficult to describe what I meant by "failing" when a family member would phone as ask the state of Florence when she was in the midst of a decline. Frequently, several conditions were being affected at one time. She would lose her responsiveness to questions or to tasks such as moving over onto her side. She would complain, through whispers, that she could not see well, and that her pain level was higher. Swallowing was more difficult than usual and feeding took a lengthy period of time. When a small volume of food was given by syringe, she would hold it in her mouth for a period of time until she was ready to swallow. This meant that one had to wait until she could get each measure down before attempting to give another. Sometimes, gently stroking her throat would help getting her to swallow. When awake she would simply stare at the ceiling and not respond to any stimuli. Once in a while, she would see color changes or insects on the ceiling. I constantly worried that she could not continue on like that without falling victim of pneumonia, organ failure, or some other terminal problem. Medication was not as easy as before. She had a major problem swallowing pills, particularly large ones. I tried liquid formulations for several of her routine drugs but the experiment failed because volumes turned out to be too great and their taste was too bad for Florence to accept. This was in keeping with Florence's basic nature of being unable to cope with circumstances which varied to any significant degree from the norm. So, I purchased an advanced electric pill crusher (*First Crush Automatic Pill Crusher*) to adequately pulverize her range of medications. After crushing, the powder could be incorporated into thick suspensions like apple sauce or thickened juices and administered by syringe as for all other food items. This procedure worked fairly well but care had to still be taken to give slowly.

By the year 2013, Florence's eyesight began to significantly fail. From the beginning she had difficulty focusing downward and needed magnification. But, once an object was in the correct plane, she could visualize it fairly well. Before a TV was precisely positioned, she had difficulty in seeing it but after a series of adjustments, she did pretty well. That too was changing in 2013. By then, it was too difficult for her to position her head just right to see the TV so she only listened to programs and rarely was able to watch them. I was truly struck by the observation that there seemed to be little life left in her eyes. They were blank as if unseeing (but not so) and no longer offered warmth or any guide to her feelings. In fact their dark brown color had faded. For me, this was a shock. I could always look into her eyes and see how she felt even when she would say nothing. No longer. I could not tell if my adjustments to her position in bed, or attempts to sit her up in a wheel chair, etc. were helpful or hurtful. Rather, I now had to interpret her facial expressions which were becoming increasingly complex. It was amazing how she had gone from hypo-expressional (expressionless) at the beginning of the malady in 2006 to hyper-expressional in 2013. I recorded many of these but regarded them as too personal to include here. In any case, as always, one facial expression was always lacking - a smile. She had either lost control of muscles that were needed for that gesture or was devoid of the necessary emotion.

By mid-2013, speech was nearly lost, and at best she could whisper words and even they were often garbled. I could still find an answer to my questions by requesting that she raise her eyebrows if the answer was yes to the query I asked. In this way, I could offer a number of different options to discern what she would like for dinner, whether she needed a drink of water, or whatever. During this period, a strange thing happened. My sister sat at her bedside one evening and suggested that they say the Lord's Prayer together. Florence nodded in agreement and then spoke the entire prayer loudly and as clear as she had ever spoken anything. It was a shock to my sister and to us all, but this phenomenon was never once repeated.

6

THE END

_____

After many quiescent months, for the first time, Florence developed a persistent low grade fever, and during the first week of November, 2013, she was much less responsive than normal. Fearing that she had once again become victim of a urinary tract infection (UTI), we promptly submitted a urine sample for culture. Results showed no evidence of a UTI. Simultaneously, she also underwent greater than usual difficulty with swallowing whether at meal times or when taking liquids, only a small portion was swallowed. The remainder would squirt out or otherwise pass through her lips. We spent considerable periods of time trying to compensate for the reduced intake by giving smaller portions, undertaking slower administration and the like, but with little if any benefit. I worried about dehydration and her weight was rapidly declining. She was very sick, and no longer could even raise her eyebrows in response to a question. Her breathing was constantly raspy and irregular. No longer could she simply cough up the phlegm and clear it. It seemed that the strength needed for her to do so was ebbing. Her lungs sounded suspicious of pneumonia to her case nurse, and in response, an antibiotic was immediately administered. She was also connected to an oxygen concentrator to assist breathing, and was given an albutrerol breathing treatment several times daily. Around the fourth of November, 2013, Florence's temperature had risen to 101^0 F. and it seemed that possibly, her first bout of aspirational pneumonia was getting underway. She was given follow-up injections of the antibiotic *Ceftriaxone* and was properly positioned in bed to reduce skin breakdown and to assist he breathing. Her temperature remained around 100^0 with minor fluctuations for the next week despite repeated antibiotic doses. Her lungs seemed to clear somewhat, but her overall condition still did not improve. She continued to rapidly lose weight, and simultaneously, body sores appeared including a bad large subcutaneous one on her tail bone which was purple in color.

From listening through a stethoscope, the duty nurse felt that lung function had improved but some roughness was heard and breathing was shallow. Florence was no longer able to move any of her limbs and was barely able to swallow. Feeding via syringe was both difficult and risky, and there was always a danger of aggravating her pneumonic situation. She laid in the bed at whatever position she was arranged at and stared wide-eyed at the ceiling. During this entire week she was totally unresponsive to any comments, conversation or most other stimuli. Her breathing was both labored and rapid (36-40 breaths per minute) and could only be brought down to about 24 bpm through repeated albuterol breathing treatments and scattered doses of *Roxinol*. We all wondered what truly was wrong with her now that pneumonia seemed to have abated. There must have been organ failure taking place in some form, but we had no way of knowing. When someone is under hospice care, there are no regular blood tests, x-rays, etc. for therapeutic purposes. Hence, any number of things may have been happening, internally, of which we were totally unaware. The only way investigate would have been to transfer her from home hospice care to insured hospital care and then proceed with any of a number of less than worthwhile tests. This option did not seem to offer any benefit since she was far too ill.

I wish so much that I knew what was going on in her mind. It had to be sheer terror for her just lying there, and being unable to move or speak. It would be like being buried alive! For a few days, her eyes were wide open with a semi coherent stare at the ceiling, hour after hour, and she was unable to speak. Surely she must have a stream of thoughts, whether good, bad, panicked or calm. If only there was a way to know, to communicate with her, to help her deal with the inevitable worries a person must have when internally dealing with the end of life. I spoke to her many times, kissed her, expressed my love and my good wishes, and once in a while she would weakly tilt an eyebrow as a sign of acknowledgement. It is said that hearing is the last sense to fail under such conditions. The hospice chaplain came and shared the Lord's Prayer, and at its end, she managed to formulate, "Amen," with her lips thus remaining strongly spiritual to the very end.

On November 12, when she awoke, her unseeing eyes only opened half way and she remained totally unresponsive. Her urine output notably increased, and her breathing was very shallow. As I looked upon her, tears flowed from my eyes. After all of the years of my dealing with her illness, I knew the

The End   104 time of her passing would eventually come, but I put it into the back of my mind, not wanting to plan or even think about what was to happen next. It is commonly advanced that when a person dies after a long, painful illness that it is a blessing. True for the patient, perhaps, but not necessarily for the survivor. It appeared that although I had plenty of warning, and plenty of time to prepare for Florence's death. I clearly had not done so adequately. No amount of time would have been sufficient! I slipped into a twilight zone, a subconscious rationalization recognizing that Florence will die very soon, but simultaneously not accepting that it would happen. I now do not believe that any amount or time of preparation would have been sufficient for me. Now, with her life rapidly slipping away, I still had no coherent thoughts of how to respond when she was gone. My whole life centered around her; our home, our family relations, our friends, what now? I thought back to incidents over the years when I was unhappy with her at times for not being more than she was (e.g., not being more outgoing), but now I know that I never totally appreciated what she was, what she truly excelled at when encouraged. Like all couples there were times when we were in a period of disagreement, and once during one of these times, she felt badly and made a statement that made me forever contrite. "I know that there are things that you don't like about me, I can only do the best I can!" upon which I apologized and pleaded for forgiveness, but I am not sure that she ever totally did. Though we were subject to occasional discord at times, we never argued. She would not permit it and simply stopped responding to my noisiness (nonsense).

The End

At her bedside during the final hours as she gasped for breath through repeated episodes of apnea, I thought back to the time when we first met. It was the summer of 1959, and I had just graduated from a small town high school in western New York State. As immortalized in the movie American Graffiti, my friends and I cruised Main Street of a larger neighboring city in my 1931 Model A Ford five window coupe. One night we stopped at a frozen custard stand and I saw an absolutely beautiful girl at work who I had never seen before. I ordered a cone from her, then asked for her name and a date. She gave me the former but did not agree to the latter. "Florence and 75 cents, please," was her response. With my ego bruised, I grabbed the cone, hopped into my Model A and sputtered away. Nine months later, during spring break from college, I decided to try again. After discovering her complete name from friends, I phoned her. This time she agreed to go to the movies with me. We interacted well and were together from then on. During the autumn of 1960, when she went to school at Buffalo State College, each weekend I would make the pilgrimage from Ithaca, New York to Buffalo to spend time with her. Not a fun drive on snowy, wintery days but I always got there. In June of 1961 we were married, but along the way I had to sacrifice my Model A Ford in favor of an engagement ring to place on her finger at Christmas, 1960. She joined me in Ithaca as our life began as man and wife and in September 1961 became a secretary in the Vegetable Crops Department at Cornell University, a position she held for two years and thoroughly enjoyed the position.

The term marriage is variously defined as ".. a legally, religiously, or socially sanctioned union of persons who commit to one another ..". Emphasis these days often seems to focus on the legal aspects of the union rather than the other elements. Sad indeed compared with those of us in which legal aspects and sharing were automatic and were of no conscious factor throughout our lives. What is not talked about enough is the concept "Wife" in a loving husbands mind. In a successful marriage, a man is proud to share his life with a person who like him, has one primary purpose, to provide, support, and care for his/her mate above all else. To make a home in which husband and wife flourish together in the presence of one another, and who raise children in an atmosphere of love. A successful marriage is a system of irreducible complexity where (according to Professor Michael Behe of Lehigh University) all components must perform in concert for the whole to work. Should any basic element be lacking, the marriage soon falters, and then falls apart. Yet, the constant presence, love and support of a wife may be easily taken for granted. Men forget that it is not easy in this life to find someone who will put up with all of the testosterone driven peccadillos for a lifetime. Only the most loving, understanding and saintly woman did so for me. For this I am eternally grateful and pray that my caring for her during eight years of illness would grant me some degree of absolution. At 2:44 am on November 19, 2013, after several days and nights in and out of a coma, Florence drew her last breath, sighed and passed away. Consumed by a flood of tears I kissed her and said goodbye. It was almost exactly eight years of affliction that she had suffered through, and it was a blessing that her torture was finally ended. Even so, this did little to assuage my pain. Hospice nurses were present to help us through it and were there to take care of the inevitable details following death. For that, we were eternally grateful. Now, I faced the challenge to find some form of meaning in my life. The first hurdle was to cease crying at the very thought of Florence being gone. It was hard to feel positive in the midst of such pain. My family gathered around and provided all forms of support, financial as well as moral. It meant very much to have them there and to remind our young grandchildren that were it not for grandma, they would not exist. Simultaneous with her death a strange, inexplicable event occurred in the home of Florence's niece, Tricia. Many years ago when Tricia was only a young girl, Florence had given her a small quartz clock to be placed on her vanity. Over time the clock was relocated into one of the vanity drawers and forgotten. For reasons unknown, before she even knew of Florence's passing, Tricia reached into the drawer and brought out the clock. The clock had stopped at the exact time of death, 2:44

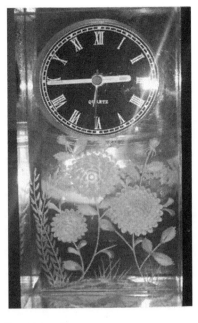

am. We propose no explanation for this phenomenon.

On November 26th I drove my daughter and granddaughter to the Kansas City airport for their return trip to Florida. With them, the last of my out of town family had all departed and now, for the first time in my entire life, I was left home alone. Wife gone, aides gone, sisters and children gone. I must now learn to go forward, somehow, and try to stay busy. I stopped at a local grocery store, bought a few goods, and on the way out purchased a plaque at the flower shop. No source for this rhyme is shown, but I thank the author for its content. It read;

Our hearts still ache with sadness, And secret tears still flow. What it meant to lose you, No one can ever know

7

Epilogue

When my father died so many years ago (1980) my entire family uttered a collective sigh of relieve. "Thank God he passed before Mom," was the universal feeling. Dad was continually dependent on Mom for all forms of sustenance including mental needs that had she died first, it would have destroyed him instantly, and caused all of us even more grief. But, our hiatus did not last long. Two years later, Mom succumbed to her five plus year battle with breast cancer. Our family was always close and we suffered through this with terrible anguish. Now, I became the senior member of the family and Florence, as my wife, became second in command. She was older that all of my sisters and was greatly regarded for her wisdom and sensitivity. And, she held a position of love and respect within my family as long as she lived. Florence is now gone and with her went all of my vitality, my energy, my opportunity to put right the things that I had wrongly done or said to her. My house was now vacant of hospice, or other aides and nurses, and it exists in a state of dead quiet, as quiet as a cave is dark. Only an occasional blare from an unwatched television set drowns the hush. While I am physically able to perform common household duties like laundry, vacuuming, dishwashing and the like, and while such tasks would keep me physically occupied, I wholly lack the motivation to perform any of them. The kitchen sink is constantly stacked with the dirty remnants of hastily prepared, uneaten meals, and the dishwasher is always packed full since I can't remember whether the dishes within are clean or not. The loss of Florence tightly grips my insides, and grief comes over me like sine waves throughout the day and throughout days of the week. If only I could stop weeping! As ill as she was at the end, Florence was still my companion and my true love to the last. She still recognized me, even though she could no longer speak. We still kissed goodnight each day as we did throughout our 52 years together, and she would move her lips slightly as if to say, "I love you." All of this once again was reminiscent of the time when my father passed away. Through all of my professional life, no matter where I was located, despite his health problems, Dad always phoned every week to see how I was doing. When he died, so did the phone line. When Florence died, so did my life line. God, I wish that I could stop crying! I venture out to shop for groceries, and pickup up far more that I will ever eat. Ahead of time, I plan a series of meals, but when the time comes to prepare them, I have neither the interest nor the will to do so.

So, now what happens? I am a typical griever and as a former full time caregiver, I have lost my job. It is not a good thing for me to simply weep daily and to spend endless hours staring at the television set. But what alternatives exist? Having been a constrained caregiver for so long, I did not have the opportunity to make a raft of friends. In fact, only one exists in town. And, I do not know how to go about the task of making friends now that I have time to do so. I have been encouraged to join this church or this or that club, but I have never been a joining type of person, and if I am to change, it must happen slowly with someone's help. I do have many interests like maintaining my large cactus collection, photography, writing, movie watching, etc., but these I can accomplish alone up without a companion.

All of these conditions are typical of a person in the midst of grieving, so say the bereavement specialists. Perhaps so, but after attending professional lectures and encounter groups, my level of anguish remained unimproved. I understand that may people benefit from any of a number of books, get-togethers, etc. relating to bereavement, and I would recommend such assistance to all who expect to benefit from such help. An excellent example is *The Grief Recovery Handbook* by James and Friedman. The authors point out that "Incomplete recovery from grief can have a lifelong negative effect on the capacity for happiness." This book should be consulted for all in the midst of grief for essentially any reason.

A second publication that I have found helpful is the small booklet entitled, *After* by The Crossroads Hospice Charitable Foundation. In this booklet, is offered the *List of Natural Responses* to grief compiled by The National Hospice Organization. Symptoms include:

- *Feeling emotionally numb and having difficulty believing death occurred*
- *Feeling Tightness in your throat or heaviness in your chest or pit of your stomach*

- *Having change in appetite, either eating more or less than usual*
- *Having desire to smoke, drink or use drugs in greater amounts than before*
- *Feeling restless and looking for activity*
- *Finding it difficult to concentrate and having trouble completing tasks*
- *Having difficulty sleeping, waking early, sleeping more or less than usual, dreaming of your loved one, and/or sometimes having nightmares* (In my dreams, I frequently became lost from home, from my loved one, from my children and the like).
- *Being overly concerned with your health, even developing symptoms similar to those of your loved one ...*
- *Feeling exhausted and lacking energy*
- *Feeling low at times of birthdays, holidays, and special occasions*
- *Feeling preoccupied with financial concerns*
- *Spending money on things not usually purchased as a way to avoid pain*
- *Telling and retelling things about your loved one and the experience of his or her illness and death*
- *Talking things over with the deceased person*
- *Feeling mood changes over the slightest things*
- *Feeling guilty for what was said or not said, or for not having done enough for your loved one* (A frequent occurrence, soon after death)
- *Being irritated with the wrong person, wrong situation, or at the world*

- *Feeling angry with your loved one for leaving you, angry at their disease, or angry with God*
- *Having difficulty making decisions on your own*
- *Forgetfulness*
- *Sensing your loved one's presence, believing you hear his or her voice, or expecting him or her to return*
- *Assuming mannerisms or traits of your loved one*
- *Feeling as though life has no meaning*
- *Crying at unexpected times*
- *Not wanting to be with people or having difficulty initiating contact*
- *Another response can be relief. You may feel a sense of relief after the death, especially if your loved one's illness was prolonged or you were fatigued as a caregiver*

While people differ in the intensity of each form of grief, it is worthwhile to understand that all in the list are commonly experienced responses and are not unique to anyone as a grieving individual. I have slowly come to understand this fact which has opened the door to recovery if only just a tiny bit.

To help perk me up, my daughter and my sister from California joined forces to spruce up my house. Kitchen, bedroom and bathroom floors were in terrible condition after years of abuse from innumerable spills, wheelchair tracks, tracks from a raft of people walking in and out with dirty shoes, etc. They elected to replace flooring and paint walls in Florence's erstwhile bedroom and transformed it into a lovely guest bedroom. Then, I decorated the walls with lovely sketches, paintings and other miscellaneous art work created by Florence making it her room by remembrance. After such generous home improvements, now, for the first time in years, I was proud of my home and looked forward to receiving guests. I also looked forward to travelling again, something that I was unable to do for many years. But, travel comes at a cost and I had been not wise enough to accumulate a comfortable retirement program over the years. I had always been too conservative during good financial times and both careless and overly optimistic during bad times which limited my ability to develop substantial retirement savings.

After a few months of sitting home alone, I decided to give an online dating website a try thinking that, in theory, this might be a means for meeting new people with aim of creating friendships, discovering companions for dinner, movie going, travel and the like. I have heard stories of success from several people and at first was optimistic of my chances for success. As a man of my age, however, things did not turn out as well as commercials would suggest. I participated in multiple dating sites over a period of six months and after having paid for the dinner of **at least** 30 different women, I came away empty. I failed to develop anything resembling a meaningful or lasting relationship or even friendship with any one of the persons I met. Some of the ladies were attractive (for their age) and, thus, were in high demand. Many would receive email invitations numbering in the hundreds. Even so, had posted pictures taken of them 20 years ago or more along with photos of dogs, cats, horses, children, grandchildren, scenery and the like, and when, at a one to one meeting, bore little resemblance to the person portrayed in the photo array. So to be successful within this crowd seemed to require any of several specific qualities (including money) that I apparently lacked. Many other men didn't seem to do much better because the majority of these same women remained active on the same dating sites for years. Along the way, several changed their birthdates to appear younger than they were. If all that wasn't enough, I found it very difficult to court only over restaurant tables, and I found this process of interacting with someone to be difficult if that was the only thing we did together. Each meeting was an audition, on my part, rather than a date. As a further impediment, I was also approached by a number of scam artists and website shills who had nothing resembling authentic credentials, and were in search of some easy money. After all of this disappointment, I discontinued such nonsense and found myself feeling the better for it. No joy in trying to buy companionship in the form of dinner (which had almost become a profession for some women). Instead, on a short term basis, I traveled with family members to places like Hawaii, Florida and New York over the six month period, and enjoyed being with family that I truly trusted and cared about.

It has taken time for me to accept being alone as a condition of life, but I slowly try to adjust and am making some progress. If I ever again have a companion, it will have to happen unexpectedly and strictly by chance.

8

References and Other Reading

Ahlskog, J.E. 2005. The Parkinson's Disease Treatment Book. Oxford Univ. Press. 532 p.

Clagett, R.H. 2011. Killing Mother: Progressive Supranuclear Palsy. Llumina Press. Tamarac, FL. 294 p.

James, J.W. and Friedman, R. 2009. The Grief Recovery Handbook. Expanded Edition. Collins Living. 208 p.

Crossroads Hospice Charitable Foundation. 2013. After. 29 p.

McFarland, N. Progressive Supranuclear Palsy (PSP) Information. University of Florida. (http://movementdisorders.ufhealth.org/for-patients/movement-disorder-information/progressive-supranuclear-palsy-psp-information/)

National Institutes of Health (Author), Centers for Disease Control and Prevention (CDC) (Author), Food and Drug Administration (FDA) (Author), National Institute of Neurological Disorders and Stroke (NINDS) (Author), Medical

Ventures Press (Author), National Institute of Environmental Health Sciences (NIEHS) (Author). 2013. 21st Century Progressive Supranuclear Palsy (PSP) Sourcebook: Clinical Data for Patients, Families, and Physicians - Steele-Richardson-Olszewski Syndrome, Symptoms, Supportive Therapies, Parkinson's [Kindle Edition]. Progressive Management by National Institutes of Health, Centers for Disease Control and Prevention (CDC). 762 p.

Surhone, L.M., (Editor), Tennoe, M.T. (Editor), Henssonow, S.F. (Editor). 2010. Progressive Supranuclear Palsy. Betascript Publishing. 120 P.

Tolosa, E., Duvoisin, R., Cruz-Sanchez, F.F. (Eds.) 1994. Progressive Supranuclear Palsy: Diagnosis, Pathology, and Therapy. Series: Journal of Neural Transmission. Supplement 42. 293p.

13406989R00067

Printed in Great Britain
by Amazon.co.uk, Ltd.,
Marston Gate.